"A powerful, riveting c
on saving lives of victin
past, current and future.

Shaunda-Lee's story has all the components of a best seller not just because she survived, but because she has this wonderful X factor that young ladies flock to.

As an experienced former police officer of over 35 years I have seen the catastrophic endings when bad things happen to these young ladies who find themselves trapped. In my professional capacity and as a friend I have had the honor of knowing Shaunda-Lee for 20 years. If anyone can get this desperately needed message and education out to our young ladies and make a huge positive impact, Shaunda-Lee has the integrity and the heart to see it through and save lives.

A Love Letter to My Daughter is riveting, raw, happy, sad and completely inspirational and every girl from the age of 13 years old and up should have a copy of this book. "

Martin Cheliak, M.O.M,
Chief Superintendent
Royal Canadian Mounted Police

"This book isn't just for daughters. It's for mothers and sisters and grandmothers. This book is for women. Shaunda-Lee addresses issues of the #metoo movement with straightforward language and an empowering attitude that bursts through the wall of shame and secrecy silencing generations of women. If you're female – Love Letter To My Daughter is a MUST READ!! "

Paula Perro B.A. Psychometrist

Love Letter To My Daughter is about guidance and noticing unhealthy patterns that you wouldn't pay attention to in any abusive relationship. In this book, Shaunda-Lee demonstrates incredible insight about abusive relationships though her experiences. The author shows resilience in the midst of challenging situations and makes this book truly educational. This book indicates the red flags in your abuser, and how the "monster" will turn you against everyone because they want to feel as if they are all you have. They don't want you feeling any type of power or any sense of confidence. This book is all about recognizing where your strength went and how to get it back. I would recommend this book if you notice these traits being demonstrated by those around you.

Nine months of loving and living with my Mr.Perfect. Nine months of covering up the bruises, making up stories to protect him. Nine months of abandoning my family and friends because I wasn't allowed and/or trusted to be alone with them. The assumptions, accusations, insecurities and endless mistrust. Then I met Shaunda Lee.

This amazing woman, within days, became my crutch, shoulder to cry on, and my final decision. Out!

Within a week of meeting her, I was given Love Letter To My Daughter, *within two weeks I recognized my life was in danger! I followed S.L.'s instructions and I was out and safe, for good!*

The second love letter 21 pages into this book, and one more violent attack. That's all it took for this woman and her book to save my life.

My decision was finalized without question, and I was out that night.

Thank you "Momma" for being my rock and saving my life!

-Read, observe and remember "No one is worthy of you questioning your purpose or self worth"

T.D.

Love Letter

to My
Daughter

Shaunda-Lee Vickery

Publication assistance and digital printing in Canada by

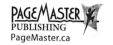

PageMaster.ca

Dedication

This book is dedicated to Braxton.
You Are Grama's Soul Beat!

I know you've got the courage inside,
And that childlike part of you that wants to hide.
Stay in that space, so familiar and pale,
Sacrifice tomorrow and today you fail
But
If you reach for your soul with strength you will find
The grips of your heart and your peace of mind.

Acknowledgements

Thank you Aunt Bunnie and Star
for their love and support.

Contents

Foreword

What you are about to read will impact your mind in a profound way. It will further change your life if only you take it to heart.... whether you are, have been, or are parent or support to a woman in an abusive situation. Do take in Shaunda-Lee's true life story as well as her first hand guidance.

I have known Shaunda-Lee for many years and her story is so very real. I vouch for her as a woman and I applaud her mission to see an end to toxic masculinity and men getting so many passes on bad behaviour that have resulted in many shattered lives and broken homes.

Welcome to your Day of Discovery!

Brynna Dixon,

MEDIAWOMYN.COM *

director@mediawomyn.com

---

*   Womyn represents Transgender women.

This book is MEATY, if you aren't triggered by this book it's not doing its job. This book helped me notice the red flags in my relationship by pointing out behaviours of my partner I couldn't notice on my own because I was blinded by love. Monsters come in all shapes and forms, mine was a mess, yet everything I wanted, and I ignored every sign because I thought it was love. I was stunned that I did not recognize red flags myself because they were so obvious.

If it was not for this book I would have focused on Miss Perfect and the relationship potential, not my own potential. Now I have a music career that is launching and the sky is my only limit. I put everything in this book to practice and I can tell you wholeheartedly that it works.

Nadine
www.arabianhunny.com

#1:
History Repeated Itself

Baby Girl,

Sometimes we cannot explain why we do what we do and when we can, the answers are complicated. What you should know is that you have the right to choose whether you are in a happy relationship or a violent relationship. You may not see that choice if you are too close or if you are scared. But it is true: You do have the power to choose. It may take time, but it is still up to you. We cannot change what others have done or what they continue to do, but we can change the way we respond to it. We can learn from it. Thirty-five years after I was taught that I was worthless, I am writing to you with the hope that I can create a space for knowledge and empowerment. It took me 35 years to unwind all those lessons, to learn who I really was, and to understand the power I have as a woman. I don't want anyone else to suffer that long, so beginning right now, it is time for you, to choose you!

Before we dive into this Love Letter, I would like to share a quick overview of my life—the events that shaped me and those that cracked my spirit. Thankfully, all those events put me right here, where I need to be, writing to you with so much love. I will be using graphic language not only because it is the language I was immersed in, but also because I believe it is important to teach you what a monster really sounds like. My apologies in advance.

Here's my story in a nutshell.

I grew up in a home, where my mother was almost murdered by my father (The Monster) at least once every three months or so. I grew up an oil brat (much like an Army brat), traveling often and living abroad. The Monster would constantly threaten to kill us. When we lived in Spain, I remember him violently shaking me awake, and throwing me from the top bunk to the floor in the middle of my bedroom. Then he moved on to my sister and dragged her out of her bed. The clock said 3:33 a.m. I will never forget those numbers.

The Monster threw our suitcases at us and screamed at my little sister and I to start packing. I remember throwing whatever I had in that suitcase, and then panicking when I realized both my mother and older sister were gone. Sucking that fear down into my tummy and choking back the tears, I mustered up the courage to ask The Monster where they were. "Gone." That's all he said. I thought the worst, I prayed to my angels that he killed them quickly, then prepared myself to be next. But the suitcases didn't make sense to me. If he was going to kill us, why were we packing? Again, I choked back the tears, and knowing my questions were pissing him off, bravely pressed, hot tears running down my face, "Where are we going, Daddy?" He looked straight at me. "I am selling you to the Arab on the boat." In today's terms: human trafficking. I started to beg him not to sell us, and he told me to shut up. We were bad, he said, and he could get extra money for blonde-haired, blue-eyed little girls. We deserved nothing more than to be a man's slaves. I knew if we got on that yacht we were never coming back. I was eight-years-old; my baby sister was seven.

The message I got growing up was that I was worthless. I was never good enough no matter how well-behaved or respectful I was, and I was certainly not good enough for a father's love. The Monster made sure to hammer this home. He wasn't much for repeating himself, and we knew any time we stepped out of line he really would kill us. I believed him. We all believed him. That threat hung over my head right into my early 20s.

As a child, I learned many things from The Monster by the way he tortured my Mother. I learned that women are to be seen and not heard. At ten, I learned that it was okay for a husband to try to drown his wife in the toilet because she talked back to him. We all knew that if we ever tried to reach out to anyone for help, he would kill us. And back then, there was no 911 to call; nowhere for us to get help.

Moving from Canada to Spain created a perfect storm for The Monster, who thrived and amused himself while he abused us. My mom, young and stunning, completely wrapped her heart around her three beautiful little blonde girls. We were completely alone in a foreign country, and since none of us spoke Spanish, faced a limiting language barrier. The Monster, who worked somewhere in Northern Africa, would skip across the Mediterranean Sea to the Balearic Islands every three weeks, come home for a week and raise hell, then be gone for three more weeks. Aside from the abuse we suffered, it was the typical oil brat life. We had no family, so the geographical isolation made it easy for The Monster to completely torture my mother, my sisters and I, without any accountability. There was simply no one to rescue us.

When The Monster drank, it made the bad things even worse. Bacardi and Coke. I can still smell it, and feel sick. As soon as the little ones were off to bed, the games began. And it wasn't just any game, but Russian Roulette—every time he drank. He turned into a complete narcissistic psychopath, and he held the reigns, controlling absolutely everything. When the craziness settled in, I watched, and I learned.

And what about my Mother? I want to shift my attention to her.

My Mother was shiny from the inside out. No matter what The Monster tried to do to her, she kept her little light shining. Whenever he went back to Africa, we got to bask in three weeks of love and fun. My Mother kept us alive, and eventually saved us all by saving herself. But the process itself took her years because she didn't know that what he was doing to her was wrong or, therefore, how to fix it. Sometimes the torture lasted for days. No one ate, and no one left their bedroom unless it was to go to the bathroom. When I was finally able to go into the bathroom, I drank tons of water. I never knew how long his tantrum would last, and water was all there was, so I drank as much as I could. I don't recall the mornings after; they are all a haze. Shock and awe, I call it. The older I got, the worse The Monster's tantrums got. The mornings after his tantrums, I found myself just thanking God that we were all still alive, knowing that when he went back to work we could all breathe again.

When I was ten, we moved to the United Kingdom and The Monster got his own office, so he never left. There were no more three-week sabbaticals filled with love and fun. The violence occurred more frequently and became more dangerous. I remember waking up in the middle of the night to screaming. Thinking he was killing my Mother and big sister, I ran downstairs to see my sister and Mother pulling The Monster off the work colleague that we had dinner with a few hours earlier. The violence was now spreading into his work. Blood—the brightest red blood—was gushing from the poor man's head onto our blue carpet: the Monster had smashed the guy's head against our brick fireplace. The man survived but he was left with massive scars on his head and face. After the man's wife picked him up, The Monster turned on the three of us. That man, my father, was held accountable for nothing—until right this minute. I will not hide in his dark, sick shadows any longer. It is time to put a hot, bright spotlight on my father, The Monster, and the horrific ways he tortured us. Until this book, and the return of my memories, The Monster has gone totally unaccountable for everything he did to his little family. But no more: I kept score.

Brave is what I think of when I think of my beautiful Mother. Strong and resilient, she gave The Monster everything she had, and still he stole more. He cheated on my Mother, then after confessing, tried to burn the house down with us in it. It was then that my Mother mustered up enough courage to pack us up and take us back home to Canada.

Things were much different back home, where my Mother's sister and brothers were. Her support system.

Family. But to me, aside from my Auntie Bunnie, all these people were complete strangers. My world was spinning, and it didn't stop until I was 27 years old and had blown through a marriage and become a sick, single mother of two.

As I look back on my late teens and reflect, I realize I was an absolute mess. I was blessed with good men in my life, a few who treated me with total respect and real love. Thank you; you know who you are. But something wasn't right. It felt wrong, and so I left the good guys and kept searching.

At 17, I landed myself a good-looking guy with a flashy car. Mr. Perfect. One minute he was buying me nice things and the next, calling me "stupid," "whore," "bitch." Then he'd surprise me at school with a limo and a picnic lunch. I was ripe for the picking for Monsters, for sure, but it all felt familiar to me. I fit. I knew my place and where I belonged. This guy didn't like any of my friends, so I hung out with his. I couldn't get to mine anyway; they were all about 45 minutes away and I had no car.

Mr. Perfect raped me. And then he insisted I move in with him and his family. I did, and ended up completely isolating myself from my lifelines, my support, my safety, my Mother. I watched this guy's mother run her ass off daily, taking care of four men. But I was there, so things for his mother improved slightly since she had me around to help. But God help her if dinner wasn't on the table when his dad got home.

I was almost killed by this guy because I tried to end my own life. Not once did I consider the woman who sacrificed her life, to keep me alive, or how my boyfriend's demands ripped her in two. I devastated my Mother. I broke her heart. I was impaired. I made bad choices. And there was nothing she could do about it. I never called her because I wasn't allowed to use his phone. So, I kept on going, spinning, dancing, trying harder, but I couldn't do enough, and I couldn't get anything right.

I started cutting myself when I was 15. After we left The Monster, the cutting stopped, but as soon as I was under my boyfriend's roof, I started cutting again to stop the hurt. The crazy-making—gaslighting, as it's known today—damaged any self-esteem I had left, which was not much. The guy was a drug dealer, and I had no clue at the time. I constantly danced on eggshells, and I would cut myself to make the pain stop. I'd do anything to make it stop. I had fallen in love with a Monster, and I prayed when I cut myself, that this time I would cut too deep.

I considered myself lucky. The worst thing this boyfriend did was rape me, but I convinced myself that he didn't mean it. I needed to be a better girlfriend. I tried harder. He would call and leave messages for me at work or on my mom's answering machine, temper lost, screaming, "Where the f—k are you? I just dropped you off. I'm coming to pick you up, so you better get your ass by that door and not make me wait!" When I tried to protest, saying he was breaking my brain—mentally and emotionally abusing me—it was all-out war. His shoving, turned into punches. I tried harder. I made him dinner. If I forgot something he would snap, screaming, "Don't argue with me, just f—king do it, you stupid idiot!" That's how he talked to me. Daily.

He convinced me that my beautiful Mother was controlling, and that I couldn't trust her. Every time she reached out to save me, he convinced me she was trying to wreck our relationship, to sabotage it, telling me she was crazy. I was embarrassed that I was being hurt and that I couldn't stop it. I could feel the stress and anxiety building, I scurried around on eggshells, and danced. I was never sure what mood Mr. Perfect would be in when he came home from wherever he had been. So instead of drowning in all those dance steps and eggshells, I began picking fights so we could make up. I would lash out, throwing things like he did, punching walls. This made me, in my own eyes, just as guilty as he was. Of course, he overpowered me. There was a gross imbalance of power and I just started shutting down. And as a good girlfriend does, I stood in front of him and not only took the bullets for this piece of garbage, I stood up and defended him. Even after the rape.

All those years of abuse by The Monster broke my brain. I believed this guy loved me. It was the only "Love" I really ever identified with. It was true love, and at 17 years of age, I was willing to die for it. I missed my graduation. I put everything on hold, so I could build him up, help him reach his potential, his dreams. I gave him everything, including my self-respect. I handed all the money I earned over to him. He was constantly telling me we didn't have enough money for this or for that. So, what did I do? "Here, take mine." And he took it. All of it. I bought him gifts, but he would buy me nothing. Loving me was a chore, so buying me anything was out of the question. I simply didn't deserve it.

I hated life, and I hated myself. I took a bottle of pills and woke up in the hospital. A kind nurse gave me a pamphlet on abusive relationships. She told me to keep the pamphlet a secret, in case my boyfriend found it and beat the living daylights out of me. This nurse was going to get me killed giving me that little pamphlet! But she was a straight talker and I liked that. No time to waste. She explained that Mr. Perfect was controlling everything and probably taking advantage of me. She said I needed to be in control to stay safe, and asked me to promise her that I wouldn't say a word to him about our conversation or the pamphlet.

I read the pamphlet before I was released from suicide watch. My head was spinning. For the first time, I realized I was being abused, and that this was not a normal, healthy relationship. I was gutted. But I was also more aware—and more afraid. It was then that I realized I was in deep trouble, and I did what the pamphlet told me to do…in secret, I reached out.

My Mother and Auntie Bunnie, where right there to catch me. The only family support I ever really had. They helped me make an escape plan, quietly and safely. They were my lifeline. They helped me save my own life. I left all of my belongings behind, choosing safety over clothes, makeup, my TV. I quit my job and went to stay with my Mother's parents, where Mr. Perfect couldn't get to me. He left angry messages. He'd call and hang up, then call back threatening me, then call back again, crying and threatening to kill himself.

The guilt I carried was heavy. I was addicted to this guy, and I wanted to go back even after he threatened my own Mother. How sick is that? My thinking was completely distorted. After about three months in hiding, I came home. Mr. Perfect had already gone back to his previous girlfriend, the one, I found out later, he had never actually left. Gutted and again feeling not good enough, I only wanted him back even more. What a crazy mess I was.

When I was 18, I worked at a music shop in the mall, and had gone to get some lunch. As I was eating my Orange Julius hot dog, I looked across the food court and found myself in great danger. I saw my father, The Monster, with his beautiful new wife (who looked just like my mother). I remember fixating on his face, dreading the second his eyes met mine. And then, just like that, he walked on by without blinking. I realized I had stopped breathing and took a huge gulp of air. I placed my hand on my heart, which was beating so fast it hurt. As I became aware of myself, I realized that everyone was looking at me: I was hiding under the table, in the middle of the damn food court on the busiest day of the week, in the biggest mall in the world. I was mortified and sick to my stomach. The Monster had so broken my brain that even after not seeing him for 18 months, I still automatically went into the survival mode I had been programmed with as a little girl. The only good part of that day was the hot dog, though I haven't had an Orange Julius hot dog since.

When I was 20 and had been away from boys for eight months, He finally found Me. The one. A new Mr. Perfect. I finally belonged to someone. In less than nine months, I was pregnant, and we were married. By the time the name-calling and put-downs were in full swing, I got sick. I was 23 when my Mother took me aside and shared her concerns. My husband was neglectful and he was mean when he got drunk. I was sick with two babies, and he was my husband. I didn't know what the heck to do.

The day everything changed was the day he went for my kid and ended up putting me in a cast. I would've left him earlier, but I had had surgeries and was recovering, and of course, there was always that voice in my head saying, "Give more, work harder, dance, and he will pay attention to you and love you more." So, I stayed. I tried one more time. Then I tried again and again, and again. Nothing changed and when I asked him to leave he flat-out refused. I lashed out. I lied. I was mean. I cheated on him, hoping that would drive him away. No such luck. I knew my brain was still broken because I ended up right back where I started, again needing help, but this time, I had two babies to worry about. I reached out for a lifeline and my family physician referred me to a psychiatrist. I was ashamed of being so damaged. Guilt was the weapon my husband hit me with over and over.

The psychiatrist I saw helped manage my medication because I was so depressed, sick with a cellular disease there was no name for, and scared. With two kids, I did not want to end up hurting myself and taking them with me in the process. Yes, re-read that. Remember, my brain was broken, so these were the actual thoughts I had.

I knew if I was going to kill myself, I was taking my babies with me; there was no way I would've left them here on earth without me to protect them. I now understand why mothers kill themselves and take their children with them. It's because the Monster is too big. My husband had already gone after my son. I know how this shit goes down. I grew up with—and somehow survived—Satan, so there was no way I was leaving my kids behind. If I decided to take my own life, I was going to drag my kids into the next life right along with me. Anywhere was better than here. My Mother never abandoned me, and I would never abandon my children. Physically hurting my children was out of the question, so unapologetically, I got help.

Dr. C saved all three of us. She used talk therapy with me. I had blocked out most of the things The Monster did to me as a child. I had no idea why I kept getting into these impossible abusive relationships and putting myself in danger. I was angry at my husband, angry at the world. With the psychiatrist in the room, I told my husband about my affair. Dr. C explained to him that I was having a sort of post-traumatic reaction to some of the things that were happening in my marriage, things he was doing to me. She explained that we couldn't figure out why, or what the triggers were, because my childhood memories were missing. Kind of hard to put a puzzle together with half the pieces missing, even if you are the best doctor ever. Which Dr. C. was.

I'm not very good at lying. I tried it and it only pissed my husband off more, which was the point. I was getting desperate, so I hurt the father of my children because there was no way I was taking him back. I loved my husband, but I couldn't respect him or trust him anymore. He hurt my child and he hurt me, I had to leave.

From the moment I sat in Dr. C.'s office with my husband and talked, he wrapped up what she said and used my broken brain as a weapon. He called me a "mental case," "crazy," "bipolar." Because I was seeing a physiatrist, he and most of his family judged and condemned me. Part of me understood: I hurt their son, their brother. But there were reasons. Good reasons. I was depressed and with the stigma our society places on mental illness, he was now armed, taking that stigma and beating me with it. He still does it. To this day he talks about what a bad person I am (typical behavior of abusive men), and he moans about what a terrible wife I was. The Monster and my husband would've been BFFs; neither of whom has ever taken any responsibility for their behavior. Sociopaths, psychopaths and narcissists are never wrong. They can be charming and sweet and in the same minute be mean and cruel.

Listen, I didn't get there all by myself. My husband was a piece of crap. I certainly wasn't going to stay in a relationship in which someone—that someone being my husband—goes off on my two-year-old baby boy because he dropped a kernel of popcorn on the carpet while watching Barney. I wanted out. Things went downhill from there, reaching the point where he threatened to kill himself if I left him or if I told my children the things he had done to me. He can slander my name, but he can't hurt me anymore. There were so many times in my life where, for my children's sake only, I'd bite my tongue so hard it would bleed in order to protect him.

But for me to survive, I needed to leave him. And like a typical narcissist, he used the children to hurt me. Rather than being a good co-parent, he was extremely volatile during our interactions. He was emotionally and mentally exhausting, abusive, and negative all the time. He was mean one minute, crying the next. Fast-forward 21 years, and here I am writing to you. It was fight, flight or freeze, and I chose flight. After an entire year of violence, threats and neglect of his fatherly role, Mr. Perfect finally met the person he is with now and left me alone to heal. But he still plays the victim, and he drowns himself in his own little pity party every night at the bottom of a bottle. I pity him.

My second marriage ended as soon as the vows were said. Even after therapy and being single for a couple of years, I still managed to pick another Monster. It was during this time that I discovered the mother bear within me. I had to pack up and leave because I would've killed the man in his sleep for hurting my child. I repeated the abuse cycle over and over, and over again, and continued to choose men who displayed at least two or three of the same violent traits that The Monster had had.

At 45, I am married for the third time. This time—because clearly, my track record was terrible—I let God choose. I couldn't pick a nice guy. I didn't know how and the signals I was giving off only attracted violent, narcissistic assholes. It came down to either God deciding or my girlfriend. She and I agreed that if I met a guy I wanted to date, I would introduce him to her first, and if I didn't get her approval (she is picky), I was never going out with him again. Even then, as a 35-year-old grown woman and a Mother of two, I still doubted my own gut. I ignored the bad vibes and made bad decisions when it came to men. Plain and simple. I dragged my babies through the mud with me, searching for a normal life, whatever that was. I wanted to feel safe for once. I wanted calm. And I wanted to stop dancing. So single it was for a few years.

I prayed for a man who would set a good example for my children so they could learn what healthy love looked like. Luckily, because of continued therapy and constant self-care, I met the man who is not only my compass, but everything that is Love. The real, healthy kind of Love.

Just as I caught my breath, I began witnessing my daughters—step, foster, and biological—repeating the cycle that should have killed me. Every time I thought I had found Love, that damn Monster showed up—in a different body, but still the same Monster with the same agenda.

Children grow up and leave, and when they all moved out, my memories moved back in. While I was trying to save my girls from abusive relationships, my childhood memories returned, laying me out cold. One of my daughters found herself in a life-or-death struggle with an abusive piece of crap, and I was literally scared to death. I knew I needed to save her, but I didn't know if I could. Just as my Mother did 20 years ago, I sat up all night dreading the knock on the door, anticipating a police officer coming to inform me that my daughter was killed by the same animal, the same Monster.

I thought I had done a great job breaking the cycle of abuse. But who was I kidding? It was as if I had my children in a headlock, running down the hallway of life, slamming against the walls, trying to get to the light at the end of the tunnel. But I failed. I failed myself, and although I tried my best, I failed my daughter.

The reason I'm writing this Love Letter, is so that every girl, every daughter—and you—can use my story to recognize abusive traits and understand how the cycle is passed down from generation to generation. I'm writing this Love Letter so each of you can empower yourselves to stop—or maybe even prevent—another cycle of abuse. When children grow up in the cycle, the deadly game continues, and it destroys people and families, generation after generation.

My love for you, My Baby Girl, is the real reason I'm writing this Love Letter. This book contains the tools necessary to help all of our daughters recognize the traits of a violent relationship before they become trapped and forever damaged. Our young women today need to know how to escape safely. We need to pass on a legacy of love, assertion, self-confidence, and self-love so we can prevent our daughters from running into burning death traps. We need to raise survivors, not victims. There should have never been a #metoo movement, but there was, and I want to help prevent more #metoo moments by arming our daughters with safe dating and rape prevention tips.

This book is for the daughter who doesn't have a strong mom, and the daughter with no mom at all. This is for every daughter from a mom who understands, who has lived it and survived, and who loves you unconditionally, Baby Girl.

I hope this helps.

Love,

Mom

#2:
Who Is Mr. Perfect?

Dear Daughter

WHO IS MR. PERFECT?

Mr. Perfect is a hunter. He is very smart and extremely charming. He is funny. He is looking for a girl who is everything he thinks a girl should be, but not who you are. Mr. Perfect usually targets easy-going, sensitive, empathetic girls and young women. He is looking for a kind, gentle person, an inexperienced, open, soft soul.

Mr. Perfect prefers girls who come from broken homes, but he will settle for a young lady who has been rebellious toward her family and her parents.

Any young lady who has been abandoned or abused by either of her parents has received a deeply ingrained message that she is not worthy of love, making her an easy target for Mr. Perfect. In fact, she might as well have a neon sign on her forehead announcing that she's looking for a violent partner. Mr. Perfect can spot this girl from a mile away, and he will jump in quickly—with both feet.

At the beginning of a violent relationship, every-thing is emotionally heightened. For most of us, there is no greater feeling than falling in love. When we meet someone we like, endorphins—chemicals that make us feel happy, light, excited—are released in the brain. Mr. Perfect counts on this. When the brain chemicals take over, a young lady will start to believe she is deeply in love, when, in fact, she is most likely confusing it with this new feeling of lust.

She can't wait to see Mr. Perfect, and clears her sched-ule, drops her friends, skips out on family dinners. She will sacrifice anything; nothing gets in the way of spend-ing time with Mr. Perfect. Mr. Perfect will convince her that they are soulmates and that he's never loved anybody the way he loves her. He will compare her to other girls to make her feel good about herself. Mr. Perfect is overly respectful to the young lady's parents, but this is part of his plan. Once her mother suspects that he is a snake and wants her daughter to leave him, Mr. Perfect will be be-wildered, hurt, and wounded because he has been noth-ing but kind, polite, and respectful toward her parents.

He'll play the victim and use her as a shield. She will take it upon herself to keep him safe and comfortable, all the while thinking that that is love. Once she is convinced that they are soulmates, Mr. Perfect will move fast. They'll move in together, convince her that she wants to start a family. But what Mr. Perfect is really doing is manipulating the young lady by taking advantage of the brain chemi-cals that are being released. Mr. Perfect is about to rip her from her home, her parents, her life—the only safe things she knows. Now it's all about Mr. Perfect.

Young women should know that love takes time. Mr. Perfect will want to take possession of a young lady as quickly as he can. Instead of allowing a young lady to focus on school or on her own potential, Mr. Perfect will paint a picture of a perfect future for them. She will follow Mr. Perfect. She will count on his potential and their future together. A normal, healthy man will support his partner in the activities in which she engages. He will encourage her to attend school and he will support her family relationships. A healthy man does not feel the need to separate his partner from her life.

When Mr. Perfect gets hold of a young lady, she will lose herself in his poisonous charm. She will push everyone and everything she once found happiness in away to accommodate him. She will wait by the phone because the sound of his voice makes her brain release the chemicals she needs to feel happy. Now, all her happy feelings are tied to him. He relies on the sexual attraction between the two of them to lure her into his web.

Mr. Perfect has a set of rules, but he is exempt from following them. The rules only apply to the young lady. Soon, she will be apologizing for everything. Mr. Perfect has her now, so he can do as he pleases. He will become disrespectful, mean, controlling, hurtful, and hold her accountable for his feelings. If they go to a family function, it will be her responsibility to make everything run smoothly between her family and Mr. Perfect, creating anxiety that she should never have been burdened with at all. When they return home, Mr. Perfect will blame her because he was uncomfortable around her family, and he will convince her to make sure that her family never does anything to hurt him.

Mr. Perfect will not assume responsibility for any actions that hurt her. He will always play the victim role, twisting the situation to fit his needs, and making rules that only she must follow. Mr. Perfect is oblivious to her feelings, and will not care if she feels that everything in her world is being discarded. Mr. Perfect will orchestrate her life to be about nothing but him, and will convince her that she must do things his way. If she does not comply, she will be faced with rejection and the threat of him leaving, which is usually enough to force her to reclaim her place.

At around the three-to-six-month mark, Mr. Perfect will expect the young lady to check in with him, but he will not be required to reciprocate and check in with her. He will expect her to over-extend herself, to give up her dreams, her wants, and her needs. He will convince her that her thoughts and her opinions should be the same as his, and he will take everything that is hers and that makes her happy, and twist it all to be about him. Once Mr. Perfect is confident that he has her, he will start to show his true colors. Mr. Perfect's intentions are to destroy this young lady using every tactic he can.

At around the eight-month mark, Mr. Perfect will have already convinced her family, her friends, and anyone who will listen, that she has done terrible things to him. He will play the role of victim flawlessly. Mr. Perfect will tell lies and convince everyone that the young lady is crazy, that she is emotionally and mentally unstable. In reality, Mr. Perfect is a textbook definition narcissist, and the young lady is neither emotionally or mentally unstable, but confused, pissed off, and hurt that he is mistreating her. When she tries to stand up for herself, Mr. Perfect will start in with the threats, the insults, the name-calling, and with time, when his words become more cruel, she will try harder and harder to please him. It is then that she will start to dance.

The more the young lady tries to please Mr. Perfect, the crazier he will get. He will not listen to her, and he will begin to respect her even less. Mr. Perfect will take to social media. He will take embarrassing photos of the young lady with or without her consent. He will record videos of sexual acts shared under the pretense of love and trust. He will hold onto these to blackmail her if she chooses to rebel. This monster has many tricks up his sleeve, but the best trick of all was convincing the young lady that he was perfect!

#3:
Protect You First

Dear Daughter

WHAT LOVE ISN'T

When we think of relationship violence, we often think of a woman getting slapped, thrown, punched, or kicked. A child getting a backhand to the face by a parent. A guy punching holes in a wall. All of these are part of relationship violence, but your brain is broken way before the physical abuse starts. So, how does it get so bad? First, you need to understand the different avenues that led to the physical abuse. And there are a few avenues, as you read in my story.

ALWAYS REMEMBER: ABUSE IS NOT LOVE.

Emotional and mental abuse ("breaking your brain") are the most damaging forms of relationship violence, and they generally start early in the relationship and worsen as time goes on. Society has created the myth that a relationship is only dangerous if there is physical harm. That's twisted.

Let's start with one of the basic ingredients of a dangerous relationship: the imbalance of power. Abuse occurs in a relationship when there is an imbalance of power. For example, if a boyfriend is bigger than his girlfriend, there is a fundamental imbalance of power in regard to size. Preteens, teenagers, and young adults may experience this imbalance of power in regard to who has a driver's license, and who doesn't, or who has a vehicle, and who doesn't. If someone who has the upper hand, in an imbalance of power situation, uses his age, gender, size, or even money against you to keep you in your place or to control you, you are in danger.

Abusers will use whatever means possible to be in control. They are chameleons. They can change their story in seconds and leave us too shell-shocked to call them out on it. Wherever there is an imbalance of power and control, there is always risk of abuse.

A boy who says he cares for you but callously hurts your feelings is the wrong type of guy and you need to get out. When you were younger, where did you run to feel better and stop the pain? Your Mother's arms, of course! That was the safest place for you to go when you were a little girl, and this is no different. You need your Mother's love, reassurance, and protection.

How can you make a difference in your life? Here are some tips.

Make Safer Choices.

Women think they are required to justify everything they do, to their partners. Your partner is not your father.

You are a woman. You have a free mind, free will, a free heart, and you live in a free country. At times you make choices and decisions out of bravery, and you need to stand by those choices and decisions. Women all over the world, today and throughout history, have died—and are still dying—so you can have the right to make your own choices and decisions. Do not waste an opportunity to make your own choice or decision.

All too often women stop trusting themselves because a guy has derailed them. As teenagers and young women, we are so awkward. We are easily embarrassed and hurt. It's not hard to take advantage of a sensitive soul because we break so easily. If you are 12-19 years old, any sexual contact you have with a guy makes you that much more vulnerable. You may as well be walking around with a giant target on your back.

Work on your own potential and your own dreams instead of concentrating on spending your life with some boy. You don't want to end up working the fast-food drive-thru window, while the boy you focused on all those years drives up in a BMW with a girl who finished school, built herself up, cared about herself, and developed her own potential (a girl who focused on herself first). Biggest mistake a woman can make is falling in love with Mr. Perfect's potential. A girl who focused on herself. Think about how that would make you feel. Give yourself time to grow up, graduate from high school. Don't expect a boy you've known for two whole minutes and who makes your heart skip a beat, want to settle down, build you a home, pay for your dental care, or contribute to your college fund. Your heart skipping a beat, my sweet, can be attributed to hormonal brain chemicals and endorphins, not Love.

SET BOUNDARIES.

A boundary is a filter you use to protect yourself, and to stay safe emotionally and mentally. Your age is a boundary. If you are under 21 and a guy wants to have sex with you, you should have a word with yourself. He will leave you, and he will take your dignity, your self-respect, and your self-esteem with him. Use your age as a safe boundary and understand that this guy isn't there to give you a Forever. Mr. Perfect is not looking for Miss Right, he is looking for Miss Right Now.

I want you to think of your life as a card game. In most card games, if you show your neighbor your cards you lose the game. The same goes for the game of life. Just as you might hold tight to some of those cards, you must exercise your boundaries and protect them with your life. The boundaries that you set should be respected by everyone in your life, including your girlfriends. A mean girl who sees your cards will call you on it. She will expose your soft underbelly, your delicate heart, and she will run with it. You should know that bullies are abusers. If you have been bullied at home or at school, you are much more susceptible to getting trapped in a violent relationship because your self-esteem has been wounded and compromised.

In a violent relationship, a guy will steal your cards and use your vulnerability to exploit you, derail you, hurt you, and keep you dancing. A violent guy uses the imbalance of power against you and it is not about love. It is about control.

Your boyfriend is not your father. You do not need to get approval from him, or justify anything you do, or have done. Keep your cards to yourself and you will be able to remain in control of your boundaries and stay safe. Boundaries protect your mind and heart.

What cards should you hold tight? What boundaries do you need to set?

Lending Your Clothes out to Girlfriends

I understand that shopping in your girlfriend's closet is fun. That is, until there's a tiff and you never see your favorite sweater again. Set a boundary. Make a choice to never lend your clothes out, unless it's an absolute emergency. If your friend persists, she clearly does not respect you or the boundary you've set, so move on. Establish the same boundary with all your friends and I promise you will eliminate a ton of drama in your life.

Divulging Past Relationships

If a guy asks about your past relationships, simply respond with, "My past is my past, and it has nothing to do with you and me right now. I don't discuss my past relationships." Simple as that. This conversation can happen on your first date or your fifth date, and each time your answer—the card, the boundary—needs to be the same. If he can't let it go, that's a huge red flag. Maybe you caved and exposed that card because you felt safe enough to share your story. If he takes the card that you exposed in the name of love and trust, and turns it into a weapon and hits you over the head with it, he's violent. If you don't get away from him, it won't be long before you start to dance to make him happy. Don't let him drown you in feelings of guilt and shame.

Let's pretend you cheated on your ex, and in your new relationship, you expose that card, that boundary.

In a violent relationship, your new boyfriend will use this card to control you. How? He starts with smooth talk to make you feel heard. And then you overshare because he wants to know everything about you. This is a big mistake. One day, out of the blue, you get a text that says, "I hope you don't cheat on me when you go to your parents' place for the weekend." So, sweet, right? He doesn't want to lose me. He loves me. A few months later, he texts, "If you go out with your friends, you better not cheat on me!" It begins to feel like an accusation. Then, "I love it when you don't wear makeup. You are beautiful without it and I don't want you wearing it because you get too much attention. All you want is other guys' attention; otherwise, you wouldn't wear makeup." So, you stop making yourself feel good, all because you exposed the card, the boundary to Mr. Perfect. His change from loving and accepting to accusing is done slowly, at first, and in small increments, but in the end, he wants you to feel bad about yourself.

It hurts when someone you love accuses you of horrible things, especially, when you have done nothing to deserve it.

If you cheated in a past relationship, it should stay in the past. This is not the new guy's business; it's no one's business, but yours. Keep that card to yourself. You do not need to confess or justify yourself to anyone. Least of all to a boy. Likewise, his past relationships are none of your business, either. It is called respect, and you cannot have a healthy relationship without it. And if your current boyfriend tries to tell you his past girlfriend is crazy, this is a red flag. All of Mr. Perfect's ex-girlfriends are crazy. This is how he avoids being accountable for his behaviour; he will do the same to you.

Someone who cannot accept your boundaries or mind their own business does not deserve a second chance. Let that one go, move forward, and work on you for a while longer.

Your Relationship with Your Family

When you're dating, your family is like an invisible shield of safety. An abuser won't bother with a young lady if she is close to her family; it's just too much work. Be loyal to your family and never disrespect them—not to a boy, not to a friend, not to anyone. Think twice before you go around calling your mom a "bitch" when she tells you that boy is no good for you. She is your Mother, your parent. You are the reason she gets up every day. A guy who wants to control you will manipulate you by using your feelings of anger and hurt to drive a wedge between you and your Mother.

Respect your family and set that boundary at the beginning of all your relationships. If a guy disrespects your family, he is bad news, and may attempt to destroy the bond you share with them. He needs to go.

Keep your Cards to Yourself. Guard Your Boundaries. Stay in Control.

For relationships to grow healthy and strong, boundaries must be established. Draw a line in the sand that nobody crosses. If someone attempts to cross that line, you must direct him or her to get back behind the line. If there is a second attempt to cross the line, remove yourself from the relationship. Setting a boundary shows that you demand respect. Protect your boundary and you will protect yourself.

RESPECT

Respect, itself, is a boundary. If you feel that you have been disrespected, set your partner straight. Call him out. Hold him accountable. Use the respect boundary you set as another layer of protection.

TRUST

Establishing boundaries is a good test of trust. If your partner crosses the line, he is showing you that not only does he not respect the boundary you've set, he does not respect you. Therefore, he does not deserve your trust.

Young female adults feel the need to explain every detail of their lives. Keep some of those cards close to your heart. Trust yourself and respect the boundary you've set. In a violent relationship, if you expose too many of your cards, you give your partner ammunition to "hit" you with as often as possible. If you give away your power, you will never get it back.

Young female adults are often under the impression that assault is only physical in nature. Being accused of cheating is an assault on your heart, your integrity, and your brain. When you are hit with that type of an accusation, your partner is establishing a hierarchy, and moving you to a position beneath him. Being hit with words can be much worse than being hit with a hand.

Your partner is not your parent. If you have to justify anything—what you did the day before, who your friends are, how you dress or the way you wear makeup—he is not the one for you. In a healthy relationship, a partner should be your equal, not your keeper. You do you. If he doesn't like it or if he tries to mold you into someone you're not, he is simply not the one for you.

From here on out, I would like to point out abusive behaviors and red flags. When you see the words red flag, I want you to immediately think of fire. You don't go touch fire do you? Of course, you don't; you know you'll get burned. That's no different here. If you notice red flags, in your relationship, you need to begin to strategically disengage. Read Love Letter #14 for safe ways to do that. Fire is dangerous. A red flag means danger.

Can you recall babysitting, or being responsible for a small child? If you saw that child playing at the top of the stairs, would you just leave her there? Of course you wouldn't, because you know that child could fall down the stairs and break her neck.

At some point in your life, you may have fallen down the stairs or witnessed someone else do it, so you understand the damage and pain it can cause. In fact, falling down the stairs can be fatal. I want you to read this Love Letter from that perspective. When you are in a violent relationship, and your parent expresses her concern, chances are it is because she sees what you can't see. And it's not necessarily because you have been blinded by Love (or more likely, a chemical reaction in the brain), but because your parent has more life experience. She is telling you to stop playing at the top of the stairs because you can fall and get hurt. Life is hard enough. You don't need to be a hero, or learn lessons the hard way. Your Mother has always put you first. So when it comes to your safety and your Mother sees red flags, listen. You don't have to learn the hard way.

I have experienced violent relationships and I survived them by the skin of my teeth. I've fallen down those stairs and I know the outcome. Your parents were around for some time before you showed up. Their experiences are invaluable and they give you guidance because they have been through some of the same things you are going through. Your parents love you more than anyone else on the planet. They are your advocates. If you bring a boy home, they will always put you first and him last. They do everything for your betterment, for your own good. If you bring a boy home and they tell you they don't like him, chances are they sense that something is not quite right. They would do anything to keep you safe and to prevent you from being hurt. When your parents open up to you, don't see it as an attack; they are trying to save you.

During our teens and into young adulthood, we build relationships with our friends, spending more time with them and less time with our parents. Some close friends become family, but that never undermines a parent's love. Teenage girls often disregard their parents' guidance and experience and instead rely on their friends for help. Seeking advice from your friends, knowing they have as much life experience as you, is counterintuitive. Your parents have been there; your friends are still trying to figure it out.

In this Love Letter, I explained safe boundaries, the imbalance of power, and how violence takes root and grows. If you are in the midst of a violent relationship, stay in control and don't panic. Breathe and keep reading.

I hope this helps.

Love,

Mom

#4:
Ripping You From Yours

Dear Daughter,

I feel your silence. It is deafening, my love. I know the self-torture of trying to keep everything straight. Trying to keep him safe and happy. I know you hurt in my absence, and I believe that is the point: to hurt me **and** you.

I am in an impossible situation and I don't know what to do. You can't hear me in person, so I am going to shout it from the mountain tops. I am going to become an expert in violent relationships, and I am going to share my Love for you with the planet. I do not give up on my kid! I do not give up on **you**. And I pray harder that your silence will never have the strength to bend or break our bond. I fill the silence with these Love Letters, so you know that I will never give up, no matter how far away you push me or how far they drag you into their mud. You need to be **you**, and you need to be loved for just being **you**. No expectations. No dancing. Just calm, safe, open, beautiful you.

ISOLATION: THE CONDITIONING OF BEING KEPT APART FROM OTHERS

How does this happen?

The most vulnerable girl is the girl who's angry at the world and who actually believes she is worth nothing. Some asshole broke her and convinced her that she was worthy of nothing, not even respect. Yes, that significant person, that **asshole**, manipulated the filters and directly affected how she saw her life. He made her believe he was invaluable, that she couldn't live without him, that he should always matter to her, even when she didn't matter to him.

I know a young woman whose boyfriend convinced her that she was nothing. He used her failed attempt to get a driver's license as a weapon against her, wounding her emotionally. I watched her beat herself up over it because he convinced her that, because she didn't pass the test, that she was stupid, a loser. Apparently, in his mind, a driver's license determined whether she was worthy of respect. There was no amount of Love that would make her stop hurting herself because she believed she was unlovable. She believed him, and his assessment of her. And how ridiculous is that? Because she believed him, she **helped** him beat her up with that twisted notion. She was already beating herself up for not passing the test, but he got into her brain and set those feelings on fire. Then he stood back and watched her burn.

There is a boy out there who will care for you, who will drive wherever you are to be with you. You deserve a kind boy who is grateful for you and the time he gets to spend with you. He'll never make you feel like you are a burden. He'll never make you feel bad about yourself for not passing your driver's test. This is the **non-violent** boy. But the boy who makes you feel like a burden, makes you feel bad about yourself for not passing your driver's test, makes you take the bus and is never there for you? He has all the characteristics of the **violent** type.

You know the type. Maybe you called and asked him to pick you up. Now you're on edge because you heard it in his voice that you are a burden because he has to go out of his way for **you**. He's pissed and you know it. So, you wait, dreading his arrival, thinking up ways to make him happy when he gets there, knowing you will have to walk on eggshells. And when he gets there, instead of coming inside to get you, instead of helping you with your coat or carrying your purse or giving you a hug, he calls from the car, "What the hell is taking you so long? Get your f—king ass out here!"

This guy won't do anything for **you**; he'd rather do things **to** you. Things he gets pleasure from, things that make you squirm and cry. He is amused by your reaction to the hurt he causes. He shares his delight with his friends and they all laugh at you behind your back. His friends won't respect you either and when they disrespect you in front of him, he will allow it. That is violence. He's assaulting your spirit, breaking your heart, breaking your **brain**.

This guy will control you. He will record your reactions in the database inside his head, and pull the information out when he needs a weapon to hurt you. He'll laugh when you cry because he's cruel. He will threaten to expose your pain on social media. He will joke with his friends about how stupid you are for staying. And then you will become embarrassed and start pushing your friends and family away. He has made you feel shameful and dirty, and you will withdraw from your life.

When a young woman begins to believe that she is stupid and unworthy, she becomes anxious in certain situations. She becomes uncomfortable in her own skin, unable to trust herself to make a decision without someone else's help. She puts so much pressure on herself, beating herself up in her head. She dances and dances like this until she becomes emotionally weary. And this is the time he will choose to strike, to destroy her relationship with her family. Because, in his mind, violence cannot escalate, if there are witnesses. ***Red flag.***

Another example of Isolation? I know a young woman who, because of severe bullying and compounding physical health issues, did not graduate from high school. She was sick and needed surgery. Her boyfriend used that playing card as a weapon against her. Instead of telling him to stop treating her that way or ending the relationship, she believed him. She was already disappointed in herself for not finishing high school. She felt bad about it before he even showed up. And then when he showed up and she trusted him, she exposed that card. She removed that boundary and in doing so, allowed him to hurt her with her own disappointment, turning it against her. He twisted the truth. He shot down her self-esteem with bullets fashioned by cruel words. A violent guy will use the emotional attachment of incidences such as these to assault a woman.

It is no one's business if you have a driver's license. And there is no shame in not being able to finish high school because of extenuating circumstances. Young women give away too much private, powerful information about circumstances that changed their lives profoundly. They knock down the boundaries they've established, or they just don't set them in the first place.

As women, we intrinsically judge ourselves, which makes us a target for violent guys who want to exploit us and undermine our confidence. Without confidence in ourselves, an abuser may be able to convince us that we are a burden, and that he is the only one who has our back. He will tear strong family relationships apart and ruin friendships because it makes it easier to control a woman.

Girls from single-parent homes are more likely to find themselves in a violent relationship because it's easier for an abuser when he only has to isolate *one* parent. If a girl's mother or father has been absent from her life, chances are that absence has already made her feel unworthy of being loved or treated with respect, making her the perfect target for a violent guy. This guy is looking for a girl he can control, one who is easy to manipulated and mold into the partner he wants, without much outside interference.

A girl will experience more arguments at home when the abusive guy she's dating begins to drive a wedge between her and her parents. He will convince her that her parents hate him and that they are trying control her by pulling her away from him. She wants to make this guy happy and she wants to be loved, so she believes him. He uses her words against her, fuels the anger she has toward her parents, reminds her of the times they pissed her off or hurt her. She becomes fixated on the arguments with her parents, emotionally stuck and unable to move on. And he takes advantage of her position, convinces her that he loves her, couldn't breathe without her, would die if she left him. And so she chooses him over her parents. But he doesn't stop there. He continues to undermine her trust in her parents. He fills the now-empty space in her heart once occupied by her parents' protection with more reasons to distrust her parents. She begins to experience something similar to the pain that comes from losing a parent, and this compounds everything else.

Once the parent-child relationship disintegrates, the young woman drowns in the distress of being ripped away from her first attachment, her only example of real Love. The guy encourages her to blame her parents for hurting her; but in reality, **he** is the one who has hurt her. He reinforces that her parents don't love her, tells her that he is her family now and that his love is the only love she deserves. He orchestrated the split from her parents and now he **has** her, and she feels helpless. This is isolation.

A thief won't steal something when others are around, watching. He will wait until he's alone to commit the offense. Abusive partners do the same thing. They remove the safety net a family provides, and insert a wedge between their victim and anyone who threatens to dismantle the little mental prison they've built. If the victim has no safety net and no one is looking out for her, it's much easier to control and assault her.

When a young woman is isolated and at war with the only people who ever put her first, it's devastating. She **needs** her parents, her family. Something is inherently wrong when a young lady is constantly on the defensive. She doesn't feel she can trust anyone, but she somehow trusts her abuser. Once he has distorted her thinking, has her believing he knows what's best for her, the rest of the abuse follows suit. And it just gets worse from there.

How does this happen? When a young woman is faced with the assumption that her family has abandoned her, doesn't understand her, or doesn't care enough to try to save her, she grieves those severed connections much like she would a death. She becomes more emotionally vulnerable, and breaks any and all boundaries she had established. Someone was able to convince her that her parents' attempts to save her were actually hurting her. She began to believe she was unloved, leaving her crippled, blinded, silenced, and ultimately, destroyed.

The young woman gets caught in a storm. Her parents, who do care, are trying to tell her that this boy is bad news. They try to tell her that she is playing at the top of the stairs. But this only hurts her because she loves this boy, and thinks they just don't understand. She places all of her bets on this guy, who has destroyed her relationship with her parents. She pushes her safety net away because she has him. Little does she know that she played right into his hand, and while he pretends to kiss her pain away, he is replacing her parents and their parenting with parenting of his own.

This guy assumes the role of parent. He tells her what to do, as only a parent should. He threatens to punish her, or worse, abandon her. He breaks her spirit, assaults the mental and emotional components of her being. He creates lifelong scars that, unlike bruises, never go away. And to protect him, she hides it. She covers it up, lies about it, fights for it.

This guy feeds the young woman lies about her friends trying to break them up. He tells her that her best friend hit on him, saying and doing whatever it takes to pull her away from any normalcy she has so he can control her.

Her grades drop and she just may quit school altogether if pleasing him becomes a full-time job. She can always go back later, right? Statistically, the chances of returning to school once she is in his grip, are rare. She can't do anything that makes her smarter than him, or happy—if he doesn't approve of it. School gives her independence. A driver's license gives her independence. A career gives her independence. He convinces her that she wants none of these things. Anything she derives happiness from will be stripped from her, bit by bit, until all she has time for is his wants and his needs. She assumes the role of protector and guardian, no matter the cost. She truly believes he is all that she has left.

By the time this isolation takes hold, the young woman is too emotionally weary to fight back. She already had to put up a fight to free herself from her family and friends to prove that she loves him, and she is spent. But she won't have time for herself. He will keep her dancing, walking on eggshells, whatever he needs so she can constantly please him. She has no time to think because if she wakes up from this nightmare and realizes what's going on, she just might drop him. And he can't have that.

A guy who feels the need to keep you on your toes, one that tells you that you are crazy, is asserting his control over you. *Red flag.* This type of abuse causes the most damage physiologically and psychologically, assaulting your spirit, your soul. A guy who imprints his lies on a young woman with a still-developing brain is altering her character entirely. This type of damage cannot be reversed.

The young woman will always experience some sort of distorted thinking, regardless of whether she gets out of the relationship. She will doubt and question herself for the rest of her life. It is crucial for an abuser to isolate his victim.

To prevent isolation, talk to a counselor or your parents; *not* friends who will enjoy the gossip. Exercise your boundaries. Avoid speaking badly about your parents in front of anyone, as this can be twisted and used against you. And do not allow your friends or boyfriend to speak badly about your parents or members of your family. **Red flag**.

Think of your home and parents as a protective boundary. You have to show respect in order to expect it. Set an example by showing respect for your family and never allow anyone to destroy that foundation. Don't give up things you love, stay on track at school, put your interests and the things that make *you* happy first. If a guy comes along and wants you to choose between your joy and him, always choose your joy.

Your parents and teachers know what is best for you, and I'm sure there are other people in your life who have your best interest at heart and who will put your needs before their own.

If you find yourself isolated, missing your parents and friends, but don't want to chance upsetting your partner by contacting them, chances are you are in a violent relationship. It will be your partner's mission to control you and to keep you and your family apart so he can maintain the imbalance of power. If he has manipulated you into giving up your safety net and significant pieces of your heart, what will be next?

Love,

#5:
YOU Are NOT Crazy

Dear Daughter,

GASLIGHTING (CRAZY-MAKING)

I should warn you that this Love Letter is a bit long. It's broken up into two parts: the first part explains what gaslighting is, and second part gives examples based on my own experiences. Gaslighting is complicated and Monsters are so good at it that they leave their victims confused, in shock, and afraid. This letter is part 1.

If my words are resonating with you and you can associate, there's a good chance that you are dealing with a Monster. I will be using the same language throughout the rest of the book and you will see how it all works together. Buckle up. Here we go!

A Monster will either pick at you constantly, or completely ignore you and withhold affection. Neglect is also a form of relationship violence. Maybe he treats you as if you can't do anything right, making you feel like a burden. And you are isolated and have no safe place to listen to your own heart. You cannot go to your Mother, to ask her advice. He wanted you to believe your Mother hurt you, remember? That she abandoned you. Your Mother is right where you left her, waiting for your call, and probably hurt because you severed your relationship with her.

Feeling so unlovable and alone is the scariest thing I have ever experienced, and something I never wanted my Daughter to experience. No one should ever feel so alone, so scared of being unlovable that she has to dance, has to work so hard to keep the peace and prove her loyalty to a guy.

Are you avoiding calling your Mother because you are embarrassed or ashamed, and fear she will judge you? Pick up the phone. Call your Mother. Tell her that you are in trouble and that you need her help. Don't be too proud to call her, or fearful that she will be angry with you. The Monster needs you to believe that to keep you derailed. The safest place in the world is in your Mother's arms. She loves you for who you are, and she will love you no matter what. If you know deep down in your heart that you are alone and in a scary, violent relationship, *call her*.

Maybe you are worried about the backlash from Mr. Perfect/The Monster. Do you feel that you have to be loyal to him because he saved you from your parents? **Please.** You need to remember that he made you sever ties with your family. He made you believe he had your best interest at heart.

The only reason you are arguing with your parents is because they can see that you are in trouble. You attack your Mother, and she screams because you do not listen. Your Mother is angry but not because she thinks you are a disappointment. On the contrary. You are anything **but** a disappointment. You are the product of your Mother's blood, sweat and tears. She doesn't understand why you insist on playing at the top of the stairs. She knows The Monster is breaking you. She knows he is controlling you. But you are not allowed to listen to her. You are not allowed to respect her opinion. You have damaged your relationship with your Mother, and that bond can be permanently broken.

The Monster has convinced you that you're hurt because your parents don't understand you, that they don't care. You are in love and you are happy, but they are not happy for you, and they are trying to pull you away. Maybe he has convinced you that they don't love you. But none of this can be further from the truth: Your parents are desperately trying to save you.

And your Mother? You mistakenly believe that she has no respect for you and that she just wants to control your life. *No.* Your Mother sees what's happening. She knows this Monster is assaulting her baby girl. She wants you to get out of this violent relationship before the damage is irreversible.

But you believe Mr. Perfect. You are gutted by the notion that your parents don't love you. Mr. Perfect is there for you; he picks you up. He *gets* you. And you'd rather keep him happy then drag yourself back home, ashamed and in need of a new start, than admit that your parents were right.

But you are in over your head.

Mr. Perfect has convinced you that your parents, friends, and extended family are bad for you. You find yourself avoiding all of those people because it makes The Monster anxious and uncomfortable. You find yourself dancing constantly to keep him happy. You walk away from the very people who love you, isolating yourself. Now, the only obstacle left for him to overcome is **you**.

Now that you have decided you no longer care about your parents, your friends, and your extended family, The Monster will make sure you no longer care about yourself, either. You see, if you don't care about yourself, it will be much easier for him not to care about you, either, giving him the excuse he needs to mistreat you. He can hurt you now and blame you for it. He will make you dance, control you, undermine you, hit after hit, after hit. You start to forget who you are, where you come from, and what Real Love feels like.

You will begin to dislike yourself, and the less you like yourself, the more respect he will lose for you. You turned on your family, disrespected your roots, your own flesh and blood. So, clearly, you don't respect yourself, either. You were easy to turn on your own parents, and he will use that disloyalty as a weapon against you. If you were disloyal to your family, he thinks you will also be disloyal to him.

This is all very confusing, I know. But that's the point; confusion and mixed signals are signs that something is wrong. **Red flag!**

If you are starting to realize what is happening, good for you. Now, pick up that phone and call your Mother because you are in danger.

What is Gaslighting?

The psychological answer is simple. Gaslighting, or crazy-making, is a *tactic* in which a person or persons make you question your own reality in order to gain control over you. It works because you don't see it coming. Dictators, cult leaders, abusers, narcissists, and Monsters use this technique to make a victim feel like she is crazy, embarrassed, ashamed, and worthless. Gaslighting is done at a snail's pace, slowly and intently, and destroys the victim's ability to trust her inner voice. **Red flag!**

Because gaslighting is a process, and one that takes time, it's hard to detect and the damage can be permanent. Victims have no idea that they are being brainwashed. Gaslighting is a violent emotional and mental assault. In order to take a stronghold, The Monster will make inroads early on in the relationship. First, he isolates you from the people who love you, which makes it easier for him to convince you that you are crazy and, therefore, begin to doubt yourself. **Red flag!**

WHY DO ABUSERS GASLIGHT?

Abusers gaslight because it makes you question your own sanity. You know something is wrong but you just can't figure it out. You blame yourself for starting fights because he's somehow convinced you, that you, want to fight. You miss your Mother and feel bad about all the pain you've caused her. You are sad and lonely. Your heart is broken because you believe your Mother left you when you needed her the most. When The Monster bashes your spirit, he blames you for his outburst: it is **your** fault he lost his temper. But he is bigger than you, and his size is all he really needs to create the imbalance of power discussed earlier.

The fights get worse. Louder, scarier. Maybe you know in your gut that you are being treated badly, and you lash out. But then you question why you did that because you were not raised that way. But what choice did you have? A gaslighter will use that as a tactic in and of itself—making it seem that, because you retaliate or mimic his actions, you are no better than he is. He will take your guilt and use it against you to justify his behavior. He laughs at your attempt to retaliate or mimic his behavior; but his behavior makes you fearful. And you should be. He is giving you terrifying little tastes of his rage, breaking you in for something bigger. Maybe when he has a bad day at work or when he's tripping over the kids.

Remember the imbalance of power? It plays a big role in gaslighting. You may not be able to put a hole in the wall like he can or toss the chair as far as he is able, but you **will** lash out so you can move from altercation to reconciliation. Starting a fight moves you quickly back into the "honeymoon phase," of the relationship, and gives you a break from dancing and walking on eggshells. You want that chemical release that makes everything feel better. Your heart is starving for Love, but the longer you remain in a violent relationship, the longer your heart will starve.

It's difficult to step back and not mimic The Monster's behavior. But if you push the emotion aside, choose not to engage, and instead observe, you can maintain emotional control of the situation. There is a difference in the intent of the violence. If you know the altercation is coming and you blow first, The Monster will blame you for the whole thing. When he is done assaulting you with his words, he may move to physical violence. He will exercise violence when he is hungry, tired or if he had a bad day at work. Punishing you feels good to him. If you are upset with something he does, you give him a reason to snap and the justification to become violent with you.

Let's say, hypothetically, that you get a call from a concerned friend who tells you that The Monster has been speaking badly about you to his friends and family. You lose your shit. You feel angry, hurt, betrayed. After all, you left your Mother for this guy. When he comes home from work, you tell him what you heard and from whom. As any strong woman should, you attempt to hold him accountable.

At first, he acts coy, like he doesn't know what you're talking about, laughing at your perceived stupidity. You feel the rage creeping up inside you, and he sees that you are getting worked up. He may try to pit you and your friend against each other, saying, for example, that your friend hit on him and she wants him all to herself. This is a common tactic and it is complete bullshit. Now both of you have endorphins and adrenaline running through your veins, that addictive high, that chemical reaction. And you bite every time.

You know your friend is telling the truth, so you press the issue. The Monster has had enough of trying to convince you that your friend is a liar and he tells you that you are acting crazy. You continue to push him and he unleashes a litany of degrading, mean, hurtful things, hitting you with them over and over, and over again. You know you need to stand up for yourself, and you do. But this time, he punches holes in the wall to try to regain control of the situation. It's a show of force, a threat. He wants to make you shut up. He wants you to cry so you can be ashamed about your show of emotion. You are sorry you believed your friend, sorry you said anything at all. You just want peace, want to go back to your dancing. He showed you his capabilities and the point he was trying to make. His tactics work and you apologize for wrecking his day.

The Monster's violent behavior sends the message that *he* is the one in control and you need to stop pushing him or he may hurt you physically. He's already damaged you severely, without lifting a finger.

Moments of rage often occur after gaslighting. Gaslighting is brutal, unforgiving and relentless. But rage...rage *kills* and you don't know what will push him over the edge, or when.

You pushed The Monster too far by pressing the issue, but he orchestrated the situation so he could use it against you. He blames you for the altercation, and you believe him because he has so distorted your thinking. To make it up to him you dance more, harder, faster, only to have him respect you less. The Monster may not have physically hurt you, leading you to doubt that you are in a violent relationship. The first time you push The Monster too far just might be your last. That alone should be enough to scare the shit out of you and make you go home.

My friend, G. pushed her husband too far, and he killed her. G. knew she was in trouble, but she was scared that she would be judged if she took her boys and left. When the boys were older, she decided to take control of the situation and leave. She tried to reclaim her life and her husband didn't like it. He killed her, and yet, he was indignant, as if it were her fault. He thought of G as a possession; not as a person.

#6:
Crazy Makers

Dear Daughter,

Continuing the discussion on gaslighting in my last letter, here is part 2.

How does a Monster cause permanent damage, and what does the damage look like?

GASLIGHTERS NEVER TELL THE TRUTH.

Gaslighters lie even when you have proof, and they stick to their stories until you start doubting the truth. A gaslighter will keep you dancing on eggshells, tiptoeing around him. His intention is to keep you off-balance so you look irrational, unstable, crazy, unable to make your own decisions. And yet, you, with proof in-hand that he is lying, believe him.

When and where are girls taught that they are not good enough to trust their own intuition, their own gut? And why do we let anyone get away with calling a woman "crazy?" Our society constantly dismisses women's feelings, but men are allowed to have temper tantrums and to put women "in their place?" **Red flag**!

You need help and you are starting to realize it. You can't go to your Mother. And the situation isn't bad enough to go to the cops—or is it? You tell your friends about the despicable things The Monster has done to you. Is that your cry for help? Your friends are tired of trying to save you and most of them have left you, which guarantees your isolation. You are scaring your friends. They try to help you but you don't trust yourself, so you don't listen to them, either. You put them in an emotionally exhausting situation, and they don't have the life skills, the experience, or the knowledge to help you. For them, walking away is easier than watching you get your brain bashed in.

GASLIGHTERS INTENTIONALLY CAUSE MENTAL AND EMOTIONAL DISTRESS.

We know that Monsters lie. And we know that gas lighters lie. They intentionally cause mental and emotional distress, and then label us as unstable and crazy. The Monster will wrap you up tight and let you spin for his amusement. The invisible rope he placed around your neck is suffocating you, killing you. He will lie, and then stick to his lie, even in the face of truth. This is deeply distressing and heightens your emotions. He undermines you, cuts you off when you speak. The more you question your own perception and reality, the more he pulls you into his, keeping you dancing on eggshells, doubting and blaming yourself. You start distrusting your own voice. You begin to question the very proof you hold in your hands, and maybe you no longer even believe your own eyes. The Monster has distorted the way you think about **yourself**.

I was helping a young client of mine break out of the violent relationship she was in. The human brain is so delicate and I wanted to illustrate how her boyfriend had distorted her thinking, to show her how badly he had shattered her belief in herself.

I asked her one question: "What color is the Sky?" She said, "Blue." Of course, it's blue, we all know that, but when I questioned her again, asking "Are you sure?" she backpedaled and became anxious like she had done something horribly wrong. She panicked. She took her answer back and started searching frantically for the color of the sky. I took her hand, walked her to the window, and showed her the sky, and again I asked, "What color is the sky?" She looked at me with a blank expression, no answer. "The Monster has you questioning your own eyesight. He has you questioning what you see with your own eyes. He has distorted your thought process." This young lady no longer trusted herself. This is the kind of permanent damage, gaslighting causes. It extends to every part of your life, making you stop living, merely existing.

The implications of that kind of control over anybody's mind can be deadly. Luckily, this young woman was able to move on and she has since found somebody wonderful to love her. But it took her a long time to heal and to learn to trust herself again. And it took an even longer time for her to trust somebody enough to give him her heart. There is hope out there if you recognize the game he plays with your head. **Before he kills you**.

Gaslighters will use Your Personal Things, Your Personal Thoughts, and Your Personal Relationships as Ammunition Against You.

This type of gaslighting starts early on in a violent relationship. While The Monster is isolating you, he is getting meaner and meaner. His attacks are random and he becomes unreasonable. His attacks become so bad that you begin to question your own identity. And this is where The Monster gets the power to make all the decisions in your life. He has created a long list of your negative character traits, and he has absolutely no problem pulling out that list and showing anyone—even your own children—and using it against you.

Gaslighters Shame You in Public.

Your Monster will take constant jabs at you, privately. And in public, he will make a spectacle of you because he knows attention embarrasses you. One snarl here, a mean comment there. He accuses you of cheating so you make sure he knows where you are at all times. Gaslighters lie and say it is for safety purposes, when the truth is, the only time you are not safe is when you are with him. Soon everything you see, feel, touch, and do is for *him*. You do nothing without his approval and if it doesn't have his stamp of approval, it won't happen. Monsters even control your food and water intake, the necessities of life. Which, by the way, is a chargeable offense.

A beautiful client of mine was quickly isolated by her Mr. Perfect. Within a couple of months, she told her family that she was moving away. Soon, she began to miss her Mother, and reached out to her. They planned a visit. Her Mother would fly in on a Friday and out on a Sunday. They were going to have "girl time," which was exactly what they both needed.

Her Mr. Perfect threw such a passive aggressive temper tantrum that she called her Mother and canceled their weekend because it made her boy friend uncomfortable. **Red flag!** If Mr. Perfect is uncomfortable with you having a sleepover with your own Mother, you are in deep trouble. **Red flag!** He doesn't want you anywhere near your Mother because she will listen to you and she will believe you. Mr. Perfect knows Your Mother can see right through him. He doesn't want her near you. He is scared to death you may actually start to think for yourself, and he can't have that.

When your self-worth starts drowning in this long, drawn-out process, he starts to ramp it up. It won't matter how smart or how self-aware you are; gaslighting can be highly effective and cause permanent damage. Gaslighters are patient and dogmatic. They whittle your self-worth down to nothing more than the dirt on their shoes.

Gaslighters Do Not Do What They Say.

If you know you are being gaslit, don't listen. Instead, watch and observe what the gaslighter does. Communication is 70 percent action. If he tells you he loves you and you've been waiting and begging for a hug, instead of hugging you, he will snap and degrade you, or squeeze you hard enough to hurt you and to make you shut up. In an instant you fear for your life. He uses his size and temper, abusing the imbalance of power to his benefit. He knew in that second that you saw your life flash before your eyes. He caught you off-guard, scared you, shook and completely devastated you. He knows you received his message loud and clear, and now he has to berate you. "There, there is your hug!" He is gaslighting you, buttering you up, confusing you. But he loves you. Love does not hurt you. Gaslighters do.

GASLIGHTERS STARVE YOU BY WITHHOLDING LOVE.

Neglect is a form of violence. If Mr. Perfect shows appreciation for something, it is like giving water to a starving puppy. Gaslighters emotionally starve you. You think to yourself that maybe he isn't so bad. But you run your ass off to show him that you are a good partner and his loyal best friend, and even with all of his broken bits, you set out to prove that you love him. But what about your broken bits? What about missing your Mother? Are you even allowed to talk about that or do you have to trash your Mother so he will listen to you? He just gets angry and you hop to it, dance! You try harder to make him love you. You love him more, do more extra little things. *Stop!* He is starving you. You are in danger and he didn't even need to lift his finger.

You are being starved of affection, starved of Love. He tells you he is uncomfortable with your Mother, and that it's your fault because it is *your* Mother. He doesn't want you to have anything at all to do with your Mother. *Red flag!* What if you realize that he is controlling you through violence, even though he hasn't even started hitting you yet? Does he restrain you from leaving? Leave marks your arms? He is killing you with his words and his silent threats. That's all. That's *all? Red flag!*

GASLIGHTERS NEED TO
KEEP YOU OFF BALANCE.

Your confusion is the goal and the purpose of your existence now. Gaslighters love people who require stability and order, using it against them as weapons to uproot you. Great instability and uneasy feelings increase your stress and anxiety, weapons he uses to make you crazy. You believe he is the only stability in your life. But, your Mother? She is screaming at you to stop fooling around at the top of the stairs; you can break your neck. You are in a violent relationship, no doubt about it. **Red flag!**

GASLIGHTERS DISTRACT YOU PURPOSEFULLY.

Gaslighters may accuse you of all sorts of things—cheating, doing drugs, not answering your cell phone because you are hiding something, for example. They do this to keep you on the defensive, to distract you from what they are doing—disrespecting you, disrespecting your Mother, talking bad about you, compartmentalizing their own life separate from you. You probably aren't aware that you are being invalidated, shamed, scarred for life. You are dancing so much you literally cannot see, Baby Girl. And you are still your Mother's Sweet Girl.

If you have a loving Mother who is involved in your life, I promise you she is coming unglued knowing that some Monster you love and trust is hurting you, her little girl.

GASLIGHTERS COMPARTMENTALIZE THEIR LIVES AND THEY ALIGN THEMSELVES WITH PEOPLE THEY CAN MANIPULATE TO PIT AGAINST YOU.

I call this tactic, "recruiting an army." When a gaslighter uses this technique, it is so he can blame you when something goes awry. Girls may sense that this is happening, but they have been so isolated and their thinking so distorted that they don't have a clue about how they can remove themselves from the situation. The people they do go to for help have either already been manipulated by the gaslighter or they have turned their back on you because they can no longer watch you hurt yourself. And so the isolation continues, and you don't get any help.

Remember when your friend told you that Mr. Perfect was out talking about you? You even had proof, right? People think you're crazy, you can see it in their eyes. You feel their energy, feel like you don't belong. Other people will believe Mr. Perfect. He will make himself out to be the victim because, look at him, doing the best he can, giving you hugs and affection. He sacrifices so much to be with you when you are such a handful, a burden. He is counting on you to feel ashamed, to continue to help him hide the terrible things he does to you.

GASLIGHTERS EXALT THEMSELVES.

Mr. Perfect will tell you that everybody is a liar and that nobody likes you. He will create such a smokescreen that people will prefer to deal with him, seek him out, not you, because he has undermined you and called you "crazy." No one would believe you now. He makes you think you are alone, worthless, nothing. You are hopeless.

If Children are Involved, the Gaslighter Will Use Them as a Weapon.

The most violent weapon the gaslighter can use against you is your children.

Mr. Perfect *will* hurt his own children in order to hurt you. He will threaten to take your children from you. Or hurt your children to light you up. And you *will* light up. Even an underlying threat can be so devastatingly paralyzing that even though you know you need to get out, you won't. He has threatened to hurt your *child*! He has threatened to take your child *from you.* A Monster is just that—a Monster. A baby, to him, is just another possession.

If you find yourself here, sweet girl, please call your Mother. Tell her you are in trouble and that you need her help. Don't let your Mother's reaction scare you from leaving the Monster.

Leaving Mr. Perfect will be the hardest thing you ever do. Especially if you are in this deep or if there are kids. You *love* Mr. Perfect. You leaving will kill him, and hurt you and your kids. You are a good girl, after all, and you have to do everything you can to make it work for your family. Your children can do without a Monster, but they need their Mother. If you don't survive, your babies won't, either.

Gaslighters/Monsters will Threaten to Kill Themselves, if You Try to Leave.

Oh Mr. Perfect will cry, tell you he loves you, beg, have temper tantrums, threaten to kill himself, blame you, make you feel guilty. And he will do this over and over, and over again.

One of my foster daughters was in the process of leaving her Monster at Christmas. He called and threatened to come to her new home and kill himself on the front step. I heard him threaten her so I asked for her phone. She gave it to me, scared out of her mind, crying, because he made her believe he couldn't live without her and that he really would kill himself. I got on the phone, told him I was her Mother, and to come on by. I told him I would help him load the gun and then make sure to have him scraped off my driveway, and then I hung up on him. My daughter lost her mind. I calmed her down, and you know what? He didn't follow through with the threat, didn't kill himself after all. ***Dammit.***

It hurts to leave someone you planned a life with, and it hurts to know you are hurting someone you love by leaving. You feel this way because you are a good person, a good girl. Monsters take that hurt and turn it into a weapon called ***guilt***, twisting it up, confusing you, frightening you into staying, which is what he wanted in the first place.

You really do Love him, so leaving him is going to hurt like hell. Be aware that he may try to twist you up. Try to keep it straight and stay calm. And if you can't trust yourself yet, trust your Mother.

You never meant to hurt your Mother. You messed up and believed a Monster. She knows that. She only wants to keep you safe. She will catch you when you fall. Don't let the fear of your Mother's wrath scare you from leaving. With your family is the safest place for you to be. A Monster will not usually take on a Mother Bear; that would be too much work for him.

When you realize you are worthy of more, pick up the phone and call your Mother. You are in deep trouble and you will need her help.

Love,

Mom

#7:
Cycles

Baby Girl,

Yesterday afternoon, I was listening to the radio, and a commentator came on and said, "I was in a relationship for about eight months and it was not healthy. I mean, he wasn't hitting me or anything, but I had to tell this guy where I went, and who I was with. It was very tiring trying to be with this guy, and when I tried to break up with him the first time, it was like being stuck on fly tape, you know the kind you touch and have to fight to get it off of you?" It was followed by laughter, of course.

Even this Millennial, hosting the show, has it all wrong. Her relationship ***was indeed*** violent. And to leave a Monster ***is*** very much like being stuck on fly tape. She was lucky to get away before it turned physical, and now she is able to laugh about it. Good for her. But her message is still backwards. She was hip deep in a violent relationship, and I bet in a private conversation you would still be able to see and hear her pain. She mentioned that she has been single since. I bet. Who wants to be stuck on fly tape?

We have already established that a violent relationship is way more complicated than just being hit. That poor radio host was assaulted for eight months she honestly thought the relationship had to be physical for it to be violent.

Sweetheart, this abuse cycle I am going to talk about is a great model and has been around for a long time, but in my opinion, it is incorrect and dangerously outdated. I need you to be safe, now, before the physical violence steals your breath, kills you. My goal is to impress upon you that violent relationships do not *start* with a punch to the face; they *end* with a punch to the face.

WHAT IS THE ABUSE CYCLE?

I mentioned before that there is a cycle of abuse, and in most of the books I've read it starts at the Honeymoon Phase, leads into the Tension-Building Phase, then on to the Outbursts/Abuse/Temper-tantrum Abuse Phase, then back to the Honeymoon Phase. And it goes on and on, repeating itself, which is why it's called a cycle. The cycles progressively become faster and more dangerous as the couple's involvement increases. That is not my opinion; that is a fact.

WHAT IS THE HONEYMOON PHASE?

The Honeymoon Phase is the best part of your relationship. All those endorphins popping at the same time. You are having fun, you feel safe, he treats you like a queen, as he should, by the way. He takes you out for dinner, for walks in the park, to the beach, you go hiking in the mountains. You are falling in Love.

Every human being on the face of the earth goes through a Honeymoon Phase in every relationship they are part of. The best moments in a healthy romantic relationship during the Honeymoon Phase create memories that carry you over the bumps along life's road. Girls in violent relationships can only pray for this, as they are being starved.

In an Abuse Cycle, the chemicals released during and after fights, are the same as those you experienced when you first met. The endorphins and adrenaline rushing through your veins are the same ones we experienced when we first started dating our Monsters. They become addicting, which is subconsciously, one of the reasons we stay. Knowing this, you should be able to separate the two and rise above the mudslinging. You want that high back because it was addicting and you were starving emotionally. The Monster has assaulted your heart and you dance and pray that he will be happy with you.

Those prayers are never answered. Why? Because there is not one conflict resolution strategy that teaches you how to survive a violent relationship. There isn't one because you don't survive. A part of you will surely die if you stay.

From a physiological standpoint, all your engines are firing good messages and the chemical reaction in your body gives you a physical high, a high that no drug on the planet could ever give you. Those chemicals in your brain are extremely powerful. Falling in love is actually a chemical reaction in the brain. We chase after that chemical and that boy. It feels good. We're happy. Who wouldn't want that?

Here's the problem. If you're in an abusive cycle of a violent relationship, the Honeymoon Phase is the only good thing you'll have to hold onto. Your abusive Mr. Perfect somehow convinces you that the Honeymoon Phases will last and that it is real love, so you stay.

There are lots of different kinds of violent relationships, and lots of different ways people can be violent.

We discussed the isolation and the eggshell dance for Mr. Perfect and how he uses the gaslighting (crazy-making) tactic. That is his pattern. During the Tension-building Phase, he uses his behavior and his hurtful words as weapons. You better start dancing, girl. And you do. You get busy trying to think 10 steps ahead of him so he sees that you are a good best friend, that you love him, and can anticipate his needs. You dance for all his hard work, so he knows you are at his beck and call.

Controlling men will sometimes ration your food and water. They withhold the necessities of life. Monsters know that it is easier to hit us when our defenses are down, and if we are weak from lack of food, water and sleep, the thought processes in our brain are affected. ***Red flag!***

From a parental point-of-view, it so difficult to see your child in this situation. This hard, cruel lesson will only get worse if you feel the need to prove you are a hero and stick it out with Mr. Perfect. Step back and look at this from a healthy adult point-of-view.

You are not stupid, as Mr. Perfect thinks. Or weak. You are a woman, after all. But you need to recognize the red flags. You need to hear the violence in his words so you can understand where you are. If you recognize the Red Flags, you will have a better chance of survival. Yes, *survival.* Now is the time to exercise your boundaries. Be smart. Pay attention.

As you begin to recognize that you are in a violent relationship, my hope is that you will be able to pick up on the RED FLAGS. Don't intentionally seek out Mr. Perfect's bad behavior. Do not engage in his rage stage of the abuse. Instead, observe. Then, reach out and make a secret escape plan. He is dangerous. If you don't know what you're looking for, you can't find it. But you know you are hurting and that things aren't right, and you are trying so hard. You are exhausted. At this stage, most Mothers may not realize that they are in danger. But if Mr. Perfect puts your child in danger, you are in danger, too.

You need to understand and recognize the aspects of a violent relationship before the physical abuse begins. Mr. Perfect counts on your shame and embarrassment to keep the horrific things he does to you secret. But you need to put a spotlight on him and expose him. You can't steal a cookie if someone is watching. Same goes for a violent person. He counts on your silence, and if he does his job well, you will keep your mouth shut for decades.

Isolation and Gaslighting are the most damaging, prolonged forms of abuse in violent relationship. And without them the abuse, the temper tantrums, the fights don't occur. I believe that the isolation and gaslighting are often overlooked, so I addressed them immediately. I believe in prevention. I believe you are worth my time, and that it is important to teach you what a violent relationship looks like, so you will know if you are caught in the cycle. Isolation and gaslighting are red flags and are indicators that moving forward with this relationship is dangerous for your mental and emotional health.

The chemicals in the brain start to die down after about six months, the time when you start to get in a groove. But now you may begin seeing things, picking up on things. Don't settle. If your relationship is a healthy one, the love will grow deeper, **not sharper**.

In a cycle of abuse, Mr. Perfect's violence begins in the Honeymoon Phase. You fight and he apologizes. He makes promises. Everything is calm for a while, and then you start to feel it. You can sense his anger, his frustration, so you start dancing on eggshells. The gaslighting starts. He reinforces your isolation, then the tension builds and builds, and builds. Then just like an elastic band, the tension snaps. And so does Mr. Perfect. And now you've entered the Abuse Stage, or Rage Stage, as I call it. After he has attacked you, he will attempt to damage your soul. It may take days for his anger to subside, but when it does, he will pretend to be remorseful. And he never feels remorseful. His actions always speak louder than his words. And by actions, I mean everything he does before he gets physical.

As a recap, the three stages of the Abuse Cycle are:
1. Honeymoon Phase; in time it shortens.
2. Tension-building Phase; in time this speeds up which lengthens the time of abuse.
3. Abuse Phase; in time will be your reality and his outburst's will go from months apart, to weeks apart, to days, and then hours, until your last breath when it becomes your last minute.

The cycle of abuse is endless, and we unintentionally teach our children how to mimic our behaviors. It is up to us to stop the cycle of abuse from penetrating the next generation, **our children**. It is time to be strong, Baby Girl.

Love, Mom

#8:
In Too Deep

Dear Daughter,

Stockholm Syndrome occurs when a captive learns that she is safer if she protects her captor, her Monster. "Beauty and the Beast" is a great reference for Stockholm Syndrome. The beauty is held hostage, isolated from her father, her friends, her life. After she falls in love with the beast, and defends him, he turns into a prince. My generation, Generation X, was brought up on this crap.

It's a fairy tale, people.

As a survivor of the following subjects, I can tell you that every single thing you are feeling right now is 100% real. When I was in school in 1990, our graduation ceremony and parties were held the week before graduation. I was going out and this older guy, Mr. Perfect was beautiful and well-dressed. He picked me up from school in his shiny red car. And then he raped me.

I couldn't speak. I was numb, shocked, hurt. I don't remember saying anything on the drive home, just sitting in his car, in pain. He drove to the curb in front of my house, leaned over and gave me a kiss as he opened the door for me. He looked at me and said, "I'm really sorry. You know it was an accident. I got caught up in the moment. Now, go inside and get some rest. You have exams to study for." I was frozen. He grabbed the bottom of my chin and motioned his head toward the open door. He locked eyes with me and said, "Now get out. I'll call you later and you better f—king pick up the phone."

I remember walking into the house, hurting so much. I was bleeding. I went from the washroom straight to my bedroom and sat on my bed and didn't move. My little sister came into my room and immediately knew something was wrong. I asked her if what my boyfriend did to me was wrong. She hugged me and said, "Yes, it's wrong. I'm going to get Mom."

My Mom took me to the hospital, and the police met us there. I went into a private room, took off my clothes, spread my legs, and let those strangers take samples from my body. **For evidence.** I felt like I was reliving the rape over and over again. I wanted it to stop. I wanted to die. The police, the doctors, the nurses asked questions and then repeated their questions for consistency. I was in shock. I was praying for death.

The week following the rape was a blur. I had to be excused from my finals, and I couldn't graduate. The principal, Mr. G., was very kind and concerned. My Mother and I went to his office to explain why I couldn't take my exams, and I sat there exposed, feeling as if I were naked. Explaining the situation was excruciating and I felt sick. I couldn't take my finals, couldn't sing at the ceremony, couldn't graduate. Part of me died the day Mr. Perfect hurt me. I was broken.

Charges were pressed a couple of days later. I ripped up my room in anger, scaring my Mother to death. Her heart was broken. She only wanted to help me, and all I could do was hurt her. She wasn't sure what to do, so she reached out to my father, The Monster. She called him and handed me the phone. "You deserve everything you get. You probably deserved every bit of it. Now be a good girl, suck it up, and stop wasting my ti..." I hung up before he could finish.

The last time I spoke to The Monster, was over the New Year holiday. My little sister and I were going to stay with him. As soon as he found out that I had gone out on New Year's Eve, he started berating me the same way he used to berate my older sister. I stood up to him and told him that he had no right to tell me what to do because he checked out of my life two years ago. *He left us*.

Not that The Monster needed to know, but all I did on New Year's Eve was drive to a different city and break my boarding school roommate out of her house so we could hang out. After I broke Teddy Bear out of her bedroom window, we drove downtown where there was a big party. The only other time I had seen a party in the street in the middle of the night, was the night The Monster tried to sell us in Magaluf. Teddy Bear and I made a wrong turn and ended up in the area of town where the prostitutes worked. I had no idea they were prostitutes. One of them shouted "Hi!" to me and I commented to Teddy Bear about how friendly the people there were. They dressed a bit risqué, but they seemed nice enough. Teddy Bear just laughed and coached me to not speak to them because they were dangerous. That was the most trouble I had ever been in. My Mom knew about it. I didn't do anything wrong, so when The Monster attacked me, I stood up to him. He had no say. And, instead of apologizing, he threw me out of the house in -20°C weather with no coat, no shoes, no mitts, no hat, **nothing**. And he stood there waiting for me to beg to come back in. **F—k that**. I started walking.

It was dark and I had no idea where I was. Suddenly, I heard footsteps. The Monster was behind me, chasing me down the sidewalk. I screamed at him to stay away from me. I woke the neighbors. I thought exposing The Monster in public would release the power he had over me. But he began walking faster behind me, mumbling under his breath about what he would do when he got a hold of me. When I came to the end of the sidewalk, I saw a phone booth. I ran to it, in my bare feet, and shut the door. I hit the zero button for the operator. Her voice, asking how she could direct my call, was the best thing I had ever heard in my life.

The operator knew where the phone booth was. She called my mom and she called a taxi with the coordinates of the phone booth. The Monster was kicking the door of the phone booth, screaming at me, saying, "When I get my hands on you, I'm going to rip you to shreds. You're dead, you little bitch, do you hear me?" This is the venom my **father** spewed at his little girl. I hope he's reading this, and I hope he knows that the way he treated his family was not only despicable, but criminal. There will be no more honor for him, no respect.

That taxi could not get there fast enough. As I went to go get in the taxi, The Monster took the cash he had in his pockets and threw it at me. The taxi driver was a big guy and kept The Monster from coming for me. The driver kindly opened the door for me, saying, "Young lady, ignore what your Monster of a dad is saying to you. Please have a seat and buckle up." The driver begins to shut my door when The Monster throws money at the floor, shouting, "You little whore, here, take my money! If you get in that car, you are dead to me! You hear me? You are dead to me!" I looked him square in the face, and as bravely as I could, said, "I don't need, or f—king want, your money! I will never beg to the likes of a man like you, the way you forced my big sister to beg, you piece of feces!" I was so scared, I threw up in the taxi. Until the week of the rape, that was the last time I spoke to The Monster.

I was angry at my Mother for calling The Monster. That was the last thing I needed. But my Mother was desperate, sorry, helpless. She thought she was helping me, but her action only made things worse.

My boyfriend wanted to meet, in secret. The police filed a protective order against him, so our meeting had to stay a secret. He told me he was scared that we would get in trouble and asked if I had spoken to a lawyer. I told him I had not. Then he hugged me and told me that he loved me, and that it really was an accident. Ladies a penis does not *accidentally* fall into a vagina. Mr. Perfect told me that following through with the charges would ruin his life. I missed him so much. His arms felt safe, and in that moment, I felt that that was exactly what I needed. The love I felt for him at that moment was as real as this book in your hands. He told me that if I told the prosecutor I didn't remember anything, they would have no choice but to drop the charges, and his life would not be ruined. He loved me and would never hurt me. It was all an accident. And if I didn't drop the charges, he would not be able to save me, or my mom or sister from the wrath of his family and friends.

I looked up just in time to see my Mother leaving City Hall after paying the utility bill. She turned and looked at us as she was walking to her car, what are the chances! She stopped to get a better look and I could feel her anger. **We had been caught!** I panicked and wanted to run, but there was nowhere to run. My Mother got into her car, angled it out of the parking spot, then sped up. At first, I thought she was coming over to talk to us, but no, it was clear that she was going to hit him. I jumped in front of him and she slammed the brakes so hard that I could smell her tires. As soon as I got home, I packed my clothes and moved in with my rapist.

This is the perfect example of what distorted thinking looks like. My boyfriend raped me. He convinced me that it was an accident, that I shouldn't press charges. He loved me, would kill himself if he couldn't be with me. Then he threatened the lives of my mother and sister. And yet, I jumped in front of my boyfriend, **the rapist**, to protect him from my mother. Totally messed up.

This is Stockholm Syndrome.

I believed that my very survival in this harsh world was dependent on keeping my boyfriend content and happy. I found familiarity and calm in the dancing. It made me feel like I was in control. In my heart, I knew he would keep me safe, that he would make sure no one else could hurt me. He convinced me that that was his job, and his job only. I thought he was being protective, but I was wrong. I became his human shield. I was grateful he didn't leave me after all I had put him and his family through. Distorted thinking.

At the time this happened, I was 17 and my boyfriend was 23. I didn't look back. I did not let the person in, that I needed most, to help me. I pushed my Mother away, ghosted her. I disregarded her fear for me. I didn't know how much I had hurt her until I felt that same paralyzing fear, that stabbing pain from my own daughters. I eventually called my Mother and apologized for absolutely everything I had put her through.

My boyfriend manipulated my total fear of abandonment, the collateral damage my father had caused. Mr. Perfect wielded my feelings over this trauma like a weapon and he would hit me over and over with it. I allowed a boyfriend to convince me that I was nothing. I gave him all of my power.

It was here that i finally reached out to the Sexual Assault Hotline at the Sexual Assault Center of Edmonton. Had that 24 hour line not been open, if it were not for the counsellors there, I would have ended my life! So I have a special place in my heart full of gratitude for Sexual Assault Centers, and that is why portions of this book's proceeds will go directly to the centers to help confused, broken people who have had their choices taken away from them, and their voices silenced, for the life time of this book!!

Stockholm Syndrome is real. It's damaging, and it's scary. I learned to be helpless. I couldn't make a simple decision without my boyfriend's direction. Stockholm Syndrome diminished my ability to initiate problem-solving abilities, which gave my boyfriend more control and power. I stayed because I thought this was normal. That's what I grew up with. I was ripe for the picking of Monsters.

The victims of Stockholm Syndrome are prone to depression and high anxiety. You are broken if you find yourself here. You are also in more danger than you think. Call your Mom. Get counseling. Your brain is broken if you can relate to this You need help unraveling and recognizing distorted thinking.

TRAUMATIC BONDING

Traumatic Bonding is an emotional attachment under the conditions of a violent relationship and is compounded by a traumatic loss. The bond occurs between the abuser and the victim, under the impact of the trauma. When we are in pain we hold on tighter to each other. The abuser, however, works to maintain the imbalance of power. He responds unpredictably to his victim, blaming her for his unhappiness. But she absolves him of his bad behavior because he hurts, too. Dance. Dance. Dance. She begins to feel bad about herself. She becomes more dependent on the one with the power, Mr. Perfect. In violent relationships, partners who are traumatically bonded find it much more difficult to leave the relationship.

Both Stockholm Syndrome and Traumatic Bonding, are so strong that even after leaving the relationship, a woman will forever long for that familiar place. And instead of looking back in rage, as she should, she will remember how good the relationship made her feel, blocking out the truth, the hurt, the devastation, hoping to, somehow, turn the violent relationship into a fairy tale.

Love,

Mom

#9:
Facts

My Love,

You are precious, smart, strong, and brave. You deserve every drop of happiness. Reading this book can be overwhelming because of the content. I wish I had all the answers. I wish I could reach in and catch you, stop him from hurting you. If you are in so deep and you are tired of dancing, the best way for me to help you, is to share my knowledge with you so you can make informed decisions, and move forward safely.

They say prevention is the best medicine. I say education is the best medicine. There are thousands of kinds of violent relationships. They are becoming an epidemic. Violent behaviors are rolled up nicely in typical Abuse Cycle models. This is important for you to know and it will help you understand if you are caught in a cycle. Here are the different forms of abuse, in order of importance, based on my own experience.

1. Emotional/Mental Abuse

This red flag comes in all sorts of forms: name-calling, degrading, blaming you for his anger, removal of decision-making rights, gaslighting. These are the seedlings you never want to take root. Abusers use accusations of cheating, meanness, neglect to get their hooks into us. If you move too far to the left, the hook will rip your heart out. If you move too far to the right, it will rip out your soul.

2. Isolation

The abuser's purpose is to set you up so no one can get to you. That is, no one but him. If you have pushed everyone away to protect him, you've given him a green light to do with you as he sees fit. You believe this is love. He convinces you that all those horrible people in your life who have been there for you from birth, were only there to hurt you. That is what he has manipulated you into believing. Your parents are the only people on the planet that will lay down their lives for you. They want what's best for you. If you push them away, you're walking right into fire. Red flag!

3. Physical Abuse

If you're trying to leave a room and a guy lifts up his arm to cross the door because he does not want you to leave, that is physical abuse. True story. A chargeable offense, too. Biting, slapping, kicking, hair-pulling, shoving, withholding food or water, holding you down by the arms, squeezing your wrists. ***Red flags, all of them!***

4. Destruction or a Threat to Children, Animals, Personal Property

An abuser will punch the walls in your home. He will use anything you are attached to to hurt and destroy you. He will make you feel afraid, threaten to take your child from you. If he does this and you believe him, you and your children are in danger. Sons will copy their fathers' behavior. Daughters will learn your behavior, and the violence will continue for another generation. This is unacceptable!

5. Sexual Abuse

An abuser will force you to watch others perform sexual acts, force you to touch or be touched, force you to participate in every and all types of non-consensual sex acts. He will criticize you for bad sexual performance. He will rape you. No means no.

6. Murder by Suicide or by Your Partner

If you have been pushed to the brink, unable to stop the hurt, which a boat load of morphine cannot fix, we self harm. We cut. Sometimes we feel that it is way easier to just end it, to stop breathing. Mr. Perfect has turned into a Monster. You feel your only way out is to die, I call it diving into a black hole. More like being swallowed up by it!

Your Monster is pushing you to end your life on purpose! So he doesn't have to do the work! If you ever feel this way know that suicide is a **permanent** solution to a **temporary** problem. He is not God! Get out!

Make a plan and leave, get help for yourself My Love. That is what you deserve. Not a pine box six feet deep in the ground. No man is ever worth, **your life!**

#Metoo

If you ever find yourself in a situation similar to that of the #metoo victims, trust your gut, your intuition. If a man catches you by surprise and you know he is going to rape you, pee your pants, poop your pants, try to throw up. Scream, "Fire!" as loud as you can, over and over. Assaults such as these, are not sexually based; they are assaults of power and control. Do your research and learn from others' experiences.

And that's the list. It is a misconception that abuse is only hitting.

The first two types of abuse paralyze us, making us feel like we don't know if we're coming or going. Gaslighting breaks the brain, and this particular type of abuse is so perverted and twisted that victims are ready to hurt themselves just to make the madness stop.

Breaking free from a violent relationship is torture, for the victim, her family, and the people who are waiting to catch her. We put everything into making a violent relationship work, when we should be running away from it. It's ridiculous, but that is what we do. Until one day, when something snaps... and hopefully, it's not our necks.

One day the victim will wake up. She will see that **nothing** she does will change him, and that she can do nothing to make the violent relationship better. The Beast will not turn into a prince; he turns into a Monster.

Love,

Mom

#10:
FIRE In The Flags

Dear Daughter,

If you are reading this Love Letter, then you know about the Abuse Cycle, and the parts of a violent relationship. But how can you spot a Monster before he gets his hooks into you? First of all, if you've seen any of the RED FLAGS discussed earlier, that would be your first clue.

Abusers are very good at what they do. They are masters of manipulation. They know how to lure you in and make you feel safe and loved. And then they rip you to pieces before you even know what's happening.

Around the six-month mark, the gaslighting and isolation begin. This gives them time to get to know you and determine what it takes to break you. They analyze your family relationships, they listen, and they take notes, so they can unravel you. A Monster will earn your trust so you expose your cards. He'll destroy your boundaries. He will use these tactics to break your brain and distort your thinking. This type of mental and emotional violent behavior is the **most dangerous**—even more dangerous than rape.

You can Google these traits; they are all over the internet. But the problem is that no one can emphasize enough that these traits are like **fire**. You do not go running into a burning building, so why would you run into a relationship when the guy is displaying violent behavior and abusive traits? It does not compute. If you stay in a violent relationship after reading this, you are in danger of losing yourself, and you may never get **you** back. If you stay, you will break, one way or another. You need to know who you are dealing with. Here are some traits of abusers.

Non-Empathetic

Non-empathetic men lack compassion, but they can disguise it with charm and flirting. They put up a smoke screen to prevent you from seeing who they really are. And where there is smoke, there is fire. Pay attention to how he reacts to someone else's pain. I was a single Mother and my second marriage was no better than the first. The only difference was that the kids were mine, not his. When that fool went after my kids, and I reacted, he had no concept of why it made me so angry. I decided to try to teach this guy about empathy, so I rescued a cat and gave it to him as a gift. He went after my kids again and I told him that anything he did to my kids I would do to his cat. Of course, I wouldn't have touched the cat, but he didn't know that. In that moment, he understood how I felt as a parent. He could **feel** my protectiveness. If you think you need to go out and rescue an animal to teach your Monster about empathy, don't do it. It didn't do a damn thing for me. He just got sneakier and meaner. I wasted 10 years of my life and, in the process, exposed my children to a monster. I settled because I thought no one would love me because I had children who were considered baggage. A lot of single Mothers believe this. But it is wrong. Children are a blessing and to have them in your life is a privilege. Your kids are not baggage. Don't let anyone tell you differently, and don't settle.

I thought that I could love my partner so much, that he would become a better person. ***Wrong.*** I let a man who hurt me, get close to my children and he hurt them, too. He lacked empathy and he could not feel anything. I wasted years trying to train a monster, trying to love a beast.

Abusers need to control everything to help them feel secure, empowered. They need to feel like they are in power because they are so insecure and have such low self-esteem. Putting you down makes them feel like more of a man. He knows you are too good for him so he has to control you to keep you. He doesn't ***love*** you; he only wants to control you. Treating you badly makes him feel better about himself. If he is failing, he wants to drag you down with him.

An abuser may be beautiful and smart, but if he has no confidence and displays controlling behaviors, be wary. Insecure men often come across as arrogant, almost blustery. There is a difference between confidence and arrogance. A confident man has no need to hurt others. An Arrogant man always will.

Highly Anxious

If he is highly anxious, to the point of paranoia, he will place extra responsibility on you: the responsibility for his happiness, or maybe the responsibility to smooth over

conflicts with your family. If the guy you're dating cannot look your parents in the eye or constantly wants to be
away from them, consider that a massive Red Flag.

Poor Impulse Control

A man with poor impulse control will throw a temper tantrum if something is not going his way. He'll
punch the steering wheel, throw something, hit the wall.
Backhanding you in the face will not be a problem for this
guy. And the first time he does it, he could snap your neck.
You don't need to be a hero or prove how strong you are.

Defective Communication Skills

Men with defective communication skills can't tell you
how they feel. By not effectively using their words, they
completely absolve themselves of responsibility for anything they say. Seventy percent of abusive men communicate with their actions and only 12 percent communicate
with words.

Learned Behavior

Men are 99 percent more susceptible to being an
abuser if they learned their violent behavior growing up.
I learned how to be a victim while I was growing up. If I
had been a boy, I would probably have been a murderer.
If your boyfriend complains about the way his mom and
his dad fight or his mother complains about how she's
been treated by her husband, run. *Fire, danger, red flag!*
Abuse is hardwired into an individual's brain and even
with years of professional help, he will never change. Not
for anyone, and certainly not for you.

Denial

I always told my kids that denial was not a river in Egypt. I grew up in a severely abusive home, and facing that truth was difficult to see, let alone deny. If an abuser was brought up in an violent, abusive home, he may view his behavior as normal, much the way I did when I was a teenager. The denial may not be intentional. You may catch someone stealing a cookie from the cookie jar, and it's in his mouth, half-eaten, he can't deny that he took the cookie and ate it. Denying his responsibility for treating you the way he does, absolves him from taking any responsibility at all.

If you pick up on any two of these red flags in the first two-three months, remove yourself from the relationship. Call your person. Your Mother. Make a plan, follow through with it, and leave. You deserve better than this.

If you have not yet experienced a relationship, learn how to identify these red flags, and don't ever settle.

Love,

Mom

#11:
We Want You Back

Dear Daughter,

So Now What? Well, first of all, you made it here, which means you are still alive and you can still save yourself, and your kids. But there is still a little more work to do.

You contacted your Mother/person, you made a plan, you put your shoes on. You took your purse, your ID, your baby, and you left. You are safe.

Expect to be emotionally rundown. You may be waffling, wondering if you made the right choice by leaving, and questioning if you should go back. You feel guilt, anxiety, panic. You are not used to thinking for yourself. He took away your confidence to make decisions with the conviction in your heart.

Rip the bandage off before you lose control and confess anything to your abuser. Trust yourself and your choices. Don't sabotage yourself. It took everything you've got to get here. Take a deep breath. You are not a dog who goes back to it's master after it has been kicked. You are a woman, a human, and you deserve more respect than a dog does, by default. That said, try to hurt a dog in front of me, you'd wish you didn't. If you go back to Mr. Perfect, he will hurt you, or worse. Do not give him that control.

Instead...

Call your person. Get Support. Go for a walk. Play with your baby. Distract yourself with healthy self-care choices. Take a bubble bath. Go shopping with a friend. Go to a movie. I remember the first time I went to a movie on my own. It felt weird, but I enjoyed the movie and I surprised myself at how empowered I felt because I was brave enough to do something I wanted to do, alone. I learned that being alone didn't mean that I was lonely. I had to learn to become comfortable in my own skin again, and it took a lot of work. But I am alive. I learned to re-love myself. I am a survivor. A warrior.

Write the storms down and be fluid when the terrified feeling hits you like a Tsunami and you have a panic attack. Breathe slowly in for five seconds, hold for five seconds, and let the air and all that stress exit your body when you exhale for five seconds. Repeat.

Calm yourself. Remember that he has caused some serious damage to your heart, your emotions. Your thinking is distorted. These moments have been programmed and now you need to de-program them into calm, self-assured behaviors. Mr. Perfect does not need to control your life. *You* must re-learn to control your life yourself.

Your emotions are like ocean waves. Those big, humongous waves want to pull you back like a riptide. Mr. Perfect wants you to crawl back to him, like a dog, like you have before. He wants you to drown in your emotions the same way you drown in the ocean if left alone to die a little more with each wave.

Write down how you feel. Put on your favorite music, and dance through it. Or get yourself a cold facecloth and a box of tissues, and a big glass of water, and crawl into bed and ball your eyes out. Tissue for the nose, cold cloth for the eyes, water to stay hydrated…and cry, cry, cry it out. You are now in a safe place and you are just riding out the storm.

Young Lady, you are a good person and leaving hurts because you know your abuser will hurt. He isn't a rock. He will be pissed, for sure. He does feel your loss. You made plans, you spent time together, and quite frankly, he had you right where he wanted you, and now that you have grown a backbone, he is pissed. He will find another weak, uninformed girl to train all over again. Poor Monster.

You don't want to hurt the person you love. Who does? Breaking up with anyone is hard, and even harder if you've spent years of your life with him. No normal human being enjoys hurting others. But you need to understand that he can survive without you, and that you can survive without him. Expect pushback because you are, after all, a catch. As adults, it should be that simple. But a violent partner will make you feel that everything you do is wrong on so many levels.

He twists the hurt you feel into guilt and around you go again. Know that letting him go won't feel good. You are a good person telling someone you can no longer grow with him in your life and you have to move on without him. **DELETE BLOCK.** You have my permission to text it to him. If he is violent, he will harass you. Or worse. So find a safe place and then text him you are breaking up with him. Be specific — do not text, call, email, Facebook, Instragram, Snapchat me ever again. **Delete Block!**

If you have gotten to this point, you need to eat. Eat eggs, salads, fruits. No ice cream, chocolate, chips, or crap. You need to fuel your body so that you can handle these emotions without your body breaking down. Eating healthy is your best bet and your second act of self-love. The first act was getting you here safe

Sleep. Emotions are heavy and breaking up with someone we love, is way easier to deal with when we are fed, watered, and rested. You have been dancing so much you forgot how to care for yourself.

For a portion of your life, you have been caring for Mr. Perfect, your Monster. As a child, I was made to feel that I was worthless, so not caring for myself, was deep-rooted in the belief that I did not deserve to care for myself. I felt out of place, different somehow. I was uncomfortable loving myself. It was so much easier to give love to others because I was undeserving of it. The messages I received as a child were wrong; I had to learn to love myself.

What is Self-Care?

Self-care is what you do to care for yourself, for your well-being. You brush your teeth, bathe, shower. This is self-care. Self-care is your attempt to stay healthy, physically, emotionally, and mentally. The physical stuff is easy. It's the emotional and mental parts that insist that you need to learn self-care *now.*

Intentionally choose to be happy. Watch comedy shows, watch happy things, listen to happy music. Do things that are fun, things you used to do, that you liked.

And if you don't know what you like try something new. You can build relationships and make new friends around something you all have in common. If rock climbing isn't your thing, take guitar lessons, or an art class. Spend more time with your baby, be it a human baby or a fur baby. Spend time with your family; they've probably missed you! I know my Mother missed me. She thought she would lose me. And being around her helped me heal.

Take your time; you are still broken. Don't rush from one relationship to the next. You will only end up picking the same Mr. Perfect with a different face. A Monster already hurt your brain. The next guy will be more violent. ***So, stop.*** You need to love yourself first. Your brain is broken, and that is okay. You didn't ask for it. It is not your fault. And now you have the tools you need to get out safely and work on your potential instead of his.

DELETE, BLOCK

It is time to rebuild yourself. With the right help and your willingness to be kind to yourself, healing will involve a minimum of a one-year-break from any relationship. You're already mourning your last violent relationship; you don't want to add another one to the mix. Especially because, statistically, you're jumping from the frying pan into the fire. Stay away from boys for at least a year. Or four. Finish school. If you are a girl without a piece of paper from a secondary school, you are considered useless. Finish school. Take advantage of every resource you can.

Concentrate on you and yours. Commit that time of healing to yourself because you deserve it. It is okay to Love yourself.

Love, Mom

#12:
Please, Help Yourself

Dear Daughter,

I know how courageous and brave you are. You made the best choice: choosing You. I know loving yourself is hard to do. But it will get easier. I know how hard this is for you. You gave him everything you have, and he still steals more.

I remember when I left my abusive boyfriend. I thought jumping into another relationship is what I needed. Thinking a new Mr. Perfect would distract me from the pain I was in and give me the love that I needed. But I realized that I was trapped by that same monster—only with a different face. I left and tried again, each time giving a piece of myself to boys who never wanted me to rise. Finally, I got the help I needed and I stopped giving my heart away to Monsters. I remember feeling like I had shed my skin, replaced it with a tougher one. Shinier, too.

Because I didn't get the proper help, I ended up marrying Mr. Perfect and having children with him. I waited 18 years for the abuse to end, to be rid of him. It affected me profoundly. Now I feel pity for both Mr. Perfect and my Monster.

Don't waste time; start putting yourself first. Be kind to yourself every day. If you learn to really love *you*, you attract a healthy kind of Love. Trust Yourself. Love yourself. Eventually, you will be ready to date again.

If you are still living at home, you have an invisible advantage. Remember when I told you that a violent partner who thinks you are too much work will move on?

Make him work. Make him earn your trust. Immediately having sex with a guy, unfortunately, makes you, in their eyes, a "f—k and chuck." That is what guys call women they have sex with but don't respect. You are better than that.

As a woman, the power God gave you is between your ears and your legs. I promise if you refuse to have sex or oral sex with a guy and he sticks around for more than six months, he is interested in *you*, not just your vagina or your mouth. He is probably a nice guy. Nice guys used to bore me. They always seemed too good to be true. But when I learned to love myself, gentlemen learned to love me, too.

Safe Dating

If you are still in school and are living at home, good girl. Finish high school. When a boy comes along, text and talk for the first week or two. Wait until he asks you to go on a date. I'm not talking about "f—k boys." F—k boys want to pick you up after 8 p.m. Maybe it didn't work out for him at the club, so he's counting on you to wait for his call, for you to be ready to jump as soon as you hear his voice or read his text. You are worth more than a booty call. These guys are the violent types. If he's a nice guy, he'll pick you up at 5 p.m. He'll walk to your front door, **not** honk the horn. Ask a parent to be around to meet him. This will put an invisible shield of protection around you, subliminally demanding this boy to respect you. This shows that your family is involved in your life. An abuser will view you as too much work if your family is involved in your life.

When my girls started dating, I walked them out to the boy's car, took a picture of his license plate, and un-apologetically looked him in the eye and told him that I was trusting him with my kid, and that if anything hap-pened to her he wouldn't make it to jail. I inadvertently embarrassed my girls. They weren't aware of the invis-ible shield I was placing around them. But they knew they were cherished.

Mr. Perfect will pick you up at his convenience and drop you off when he is done with you. He will tell you he is uncomfortable and anxious around your parents, dumping the responsibility for his happiness on you. He will not look your parents in the eye because your parents know he is not good for you. **Red flags!**

A bad boy's behavior is just as telling as a boy's good behavior, if you know what to look for. And if you are not having sex with him, it will be easier to let him go. Your vagina and your body, are gifts. They are to be respected. They are not to be given up unless the guy you are dating has put in the time to make it emotionally safe for you to let him in. A month or two of dating is not enough time to establish that emotional safety. If you have sex too early in a relationship, you will lose the respect of the guy you are dating. Make him wait. If he doesn't like it, too bad. It means that he is simply not the right kind of guy for you. If he is pushy, it means that he is violent. Move on.

If you want to kiss and make out, get him to park somewhere familiar, like your own backyard.. Do not let a guy you hardly know take you out in the middle of nowhere, where you are vulnerable and have no way out. Always put your safety first.

If you realize after a couple of months, that he is not for you, or if you have seen some *red flags*, end the relationship on your doorstep; don't let him take you somewhere secluded. He will have an emotional reaction, so you need to be somewhere you feel safe. Be kind, be assertive, get to the point, rip the bandage off, say goodbye, and walk right back into your own home. This avoids an awkward ride home if he is a nice guy. If he displayed *red flags*, the worst thing you can do is go to some secluded spot so you can hurt his feelings. You don't know how he will react when you reject him, even if you do it nicely. A simple breakup can turn ugly and dangerous in a split second. If you are at home, on your own doorstep, you will have power and your family will be nearby if you need support. Plan it beforehand. Your parents will gladly be there for you with that invisible, protective shield. Let your parents be a part of keeping you safe.

When you end the relationship, you don't need to justify yourself or let him down easy. Tell him it isn't working for you. Tell him you cannot continue seeing him. That's it. That's all you need to say. Saying anything else will just make what already feels bad, feel worse. It is not your job to make him feel better.

CURFEWS

Growing up, I hated curfews. I felt like my parents wanted to control everything, including my time. **Wrong.** That is a typical girl response to a curfew. Most parents need some advice when it comes to curfews because most of us parents did not know how to explain it. Well here it is.

A curfew is put in place to maintain the protective shield, forcing boys to respect you. It is also a timeline in case anything were to happen to you. If you were supposed to be home at 11 p.m. and you don't show, the authorities will have a timeline. Curfews are put in place to protect you. It is a dangerous world out there, not just because of the Monsters in our lives, but because there are Monsters everywhere.

This is an issue close to my heart. **My own father tried to sell me.** Human trafficking is at an all-time high. Girls go missing from schools, malls, right off the street. One minute they are walking along with their faces in their cell phones, music blaring in their ears, completely unaware of their surroundings, and the next minute they are gone. Respect your curfew and stop giving your parents a bloody headache. The curfew is there for **your** safety.

If you are a young lady and you enjoy going to nightclubs, always go with friends. Never go alone. Ever. If you meet a guy and he wants to hang out after the bar closes, this should be a **red flag.** Stay with your friends and be aware of your surroundings. Tell the guy that he needs to date you for a while before you will sleep with him. Tell him if he wants to see you again, he is going to have to take you on a real date because you don't know yet if you like him or not. You are demanding respect. Chances are, if he's a nice guy, he will show up, take you to dinner and get to know you—what is between your ears and **not** what is between your legs.

Safety is very important. The rules of relationships have changed. Women are more liberal with their bodies, but sex too early in a relationship, even if he is a nice guy, can diminish the respect he has for you. He needs to earn that privilege. The longer you make him wait, the more he will want you. If he is a Monster or a beast or even Mr. Perfect, he will view you as a cheap f—k and chuck, and you will never have the chance to earn that respect back. It will only create an imbalance of power, which is not a healthy way to start a relationship. If your relationship is built on a foundation of sex, how do you expect it to be a healthy relationship? Set yourself up for success by protecting your dignity. Practice self-care. Put those boundaries up and stick to them.

There are safe dating resources everywhere. Use them to keep yourself safe. You are an intelligent, strong woman; act like it. Acknowledge those **red flags**, and respect yourself enough to move away from them. Love yourself, get help. Love your babies. Protect them. Move on.

PREVENTION

My Love, thank you for taking the time to read this book. I have been right where you are. When that nurse came to me in the hospital and gave me that pamphlet, I went right back to Mr. Perfect. But reading that pamphlet, gave me the knowledge and ability to start recognizing the violent traits in Mr. Perfect. I called my Mother and my Aunt in secret, and I made a plan to escape safely. I did not involve Mr. Perfect; I kept the plan to myself. That was the very first time I empowered myself. It felt good.

After you leave, be kind to yourself. Set up a meeting with a counselor and give your brain the care it needs. Do not invest in another boy because you think it is easier to leave Mr. Perfect if you have someone else waiting for you. The decision-making part of your brain is still developing until you are 25 years old and a Monster will impair the way you look at yourself. If you continue to neglect yourself, you will break. Jumping right into another relationship is dangerous. A Monster has already molded you to conform to his wishes, making it easier for another guy to jump in and derail you further.

I am proud of you. You are a good girl, and a good person. You are loved and cherished. You mean everything to me. You mean everything to God. My job as a Mother is to teach you these things. These words are covered in Light and Love for your ears only. Stay safe, and come home to heal and reset. You are missed terribly. And, My Love, if you refuse to hear my love, my warning, I am going to shout it from the mountain tops until you come home. That is a promise. I don't let my kids fall through the cracks. I won't let you fall. I will catch you every time.

Love always and forever

Mom

XOXOXOXOXOXOXOXOXOXOXO

#13:
From the Outside

If you have a daughter or a friend who is experiencing mental, emotional, and/or physical abuse, please understand that she will push you away by any means possible so that Mr. Perfect is comfortable with her isolation. If you are like me, it's devastating.

I believe the only reason my daughters survived these relationships is because I told them the truth about what I saw and thought, and reminded them often that they matter and that I would always be right where they left me. No matter how disrespectful cruel they were, I drew the line and did not waffle. The average time it takes to pull a daughter or a friend out of an abusive situation, especially if there are children involved, can be as long as three years.

There will be times where you will be tested and there will be times when you are in the middle of the floor screaming at God to take care of your little girl and your grandchildren because Mr. Perfect will be in complete control. He will slander her to his family and friends, and the small town he grew up in will swallow her whole. He is a planner and if he can control her through the court system or through fear, you will do whatever it takes to keep the peace. She will call you in shock and tell you everything he is doing to hurt her. You must stay calm and respect her choices. In the same breath, your daughter or friend will defend Mr. Perfect and blame herself. Tell her you love her—no matter what! Even if she ghosts you, you must keep that line of communication open so you can gather your village to help support her. Send an I love You text every week or a nice little inspirational photo that tells your child that she is important and deserves better, and that you're ready to catch her when she's ready to jump.

I planned ahead for my daughter so she had a place to go and someone to support her. If you're being isolated from your daughter and your grandchildren you can be damn sure that Mr. Perfect is hurting them, controlling her, and smiling at his own evilness. Everyone around Mr. Perfect will be smug and proud of themselves for destroying the little girl you spent your whole heart raising. You need to be patient and continue with that unconditional love, and sometimes, you will just have to bite your tongue and listen. Continue positive affirmations and love her even when she exhausts you. Many friends will walk away from a young lady caught in the cycle because it is so difficult to support a friend repeatedly. It is taxing emotionally for everyone who touches her life. Gather as much information about relationship violence as you can and help her make a contingency plan. Be consistent, be steady, and be ready to help her escape no matter how long it takes. Why? Because it is so much better than planning her funeral.

I wrote this book to save our daughters.

I wrote this book because the systems **still** favors the criminal and **not** the young lady seeking protection. Primary caregivers are being persecuted the same way I was 25 years ago and the only way to stop the bleeding is through **prevention**.

There are parents out there suffering because a Monster took their baby, isolated her, and pushed her so far that she had no other choice than to take her own life. That is what Monsters want. It is up to us to never give up, to not believe the lies, and to be loyal our daughters **no matter what**. Fight back, stand up, and save your daughter's life by sharing my story.

Prevention is the **only** way!

I pray for you as you read this. I understand the pain, and the constant fear and anger. You are not alone. You matter. Your baby matters. I see you and I pray you heal from all the trauma you relive.

God save our daughters!

Best Regards,
Shaunda-Lee Vickery

#14:
The Plan

The safest plan should be formed in complete secret with only key people in your life knowing about it. And if you have children with a Monster who is using them as a weapon to hurt you, you better believe your babies are in more danger then you. Why? Because they are little and break easily.

A Monster—Mr. Perfect—uses your child as a weapon to hurt you. The best way to hurt and control you is by hurting your heart, and all Monsters know the way to do this is through your children. It doesn't matter if this is your baby's father or a new boyfriend. Male tigers and lions eat their young. That is nature. If Mr. Perfect is emotionally, mentally, or physically abusive to you, he will be the same way with your children. That is how the cycle works. He spreads his evil by inconveniencing you and using the children as a control tactic.

I remember the very first time I went out with my girlfriends about six months after My Beautiful Baby Boy was born. I got home around midnight. When my son woke up early the next morning, I asked Mr. Perfect to get up with the baby. His response was, "Too bad! You wanted to go out and have fun, so you will get up and you will look after the baby!" He didn't care if I was tired or if I was sick, the kids were my job.

After I left Mr. Perfect, he would purposefully stand our kids up on his weekends so I could not go out with my friends. He used the kids as a control tactic, not realizing it was the kids that he was hurting. There was no co-parenting; all he wanted to do was hurt me, using the kids as a weapon to do so. He continues to do this still because I left him, and the kids were his only way to hurt me.

I have seen some fathers walk right out the door with the baby, without warning, and without any contact information. The legal process to get a baby back is difficult for women, who must get legal representation by appealing to the courts. And even then, visitation is ordered by the court. Many young women can't handle the trauma of a Monster taking their babies. The pain is so great, that suicide feels like the only way to escape the pain. But that is the point—to hurt them by using the baby as a weapon.

Another young mother I know was beaten severely, followed by the children's father beating and murdering his own children in front of their mother. He happily went to jail, leaving the mother barely alive so she would forever remember watching her two children being beat to death by their father. Mr. Perfect really is a Monster.

If Mr. Perfect attacks you verbally in front of your kids, the abuse is damaging to your children. Now that you have a better understanding of Relationship Violence, you know that your child is watching the abuse and that you are willfully exposing your child to abuse, making you just at fault as Mr. Perfect. You really need to have a safe plan, a safe exit, and you need to get started right now because the damage and trauma is causing your children unrepairable damage. For reference, visit YouTube and find "Lisa's 911 Call". Force yourself to listen to the whole thing and understand that your child experiences the same terror as Lisa.

Forming a plan is daunting since you're probably physically and emotionally exhausted from being battered and suffering brain trauma. This is where you must dig deep because the steps in the plan take courage and the kind of bravery that instinctually begin as a survival tool—*flight!*

What does the plan look like?

1. Make sure to prepare yourself emotionally and physically. Sleep, eat, stay hydrated and practice self-care so your thinking and emotional responses are normal. When you start this journey, there is no turning back. Sixty-five percent of young women who go back to Mr. Perfect risk not only losing their lives to Mr. Perfect, but also risk him pushing them so far that they choose to take their own lives. Women who harm themselves give Mr. Perfect the ultimate satisfaction because he will not be charged with murder. Suicide is not an option—it is only a permanent solution to a temporary problem.

2. Start saving money and hiding it. Get the phone numbers of the women's shelters and social services in your new destination. Wrap your head around the fact that you are going to have to leave everything, but that that is okay because things are replaceable; *you* are not.

3. Get your map out and find a place that will make it very difficult for Mr. perfect to get to you. Some young women have moved across oceans and mountains to get away and save themselves and their children. Once you leave, Mr. Perfect is no longer the one in control—*you* are. It may be tempting to want to confide in someone, but it is best to keep this to yourself.

4. Pick the destination look at the rental properties and explore the jobs so you can support yourself. Make arrangements so you have a safe place to run to.

5. Sneak out when Mr. Perfect is at work. Cancel your phone number and all your social media. Delete all apps and stay off of them for at least one year. This will take a lot of willpower, but your life and your future are in the balance. In my experience, Monsters have found women through social media, resulting in severe punishment or death. Once you've settled down in your new destination you can create new accounts but you have to let Mr. Perfect become exhausted. The harder it is for him to find you, the quicker he gets bored and if he hasn't already lined up a new victim, he will find one.

6. When you get to your destination, get connected with a therapist. When you break your teeth you go to a dentist, when you break a bone you go to an orthopaedic surgeon, when someone has damaged and broken your brain and the way you see yourself, then you go to a counselor, psychiatrist, or a therapist. Consistency is the key here so make sure that you get in to see somebody as fast as possible and see them weekly for at least six months. This also takes a lot of

courage and energy, but you are worth it. Make that commitment and stick to it.

7. ***Never go back!*** If you break one of these guidelines, Mr. Perfect will find you. One young woman told me that she got into trouble because she was screaming during an episode of abuse. Mr. Perfect put a pillow over her face to quiet her so their neighbors wouldn't hear the torture, and call the police. He told her he wouldn't have to smoother her if she didn't scream. When Mr. Perfect was holding that pillow over her face, he was only getting a taste of what it felt like to kill her. Some women die when Mr. Perfect leaves that pillow on their face just a couple of seconds too long. "Accidents" happen.

8. When you get to your destination go to the police and get a protection order for you and your child if you are a mother. Ask the police to keep your new contact information silent because you fear for your life and your mental, emotional and physical wellbeing. Getting a protection order should only take about a week from the time you arrive at your new destination.

Make your plan and make it airtight. When you get scared of jumping and running for your life, stop and remind yourself that ***you*** matter. And if you have a child or children, ***their*** lives matter, too! All Mr. Perfect's lies, gossip, and character assassination are used to keep you under his thumb. If you do not remove yourself from the situation and stay hidden or as far away as possible, you are only risking your life further.

There is no time to waste—get started ***now!***

Best Regards,
Shaunda-Lee Vickery

About the Author

When Shaunda-Lee was a child living in Mallorca Spain. She watched her Mother take in an Iranian Princess to hide and protect and care for during the Iranian coup in the early 1980s. This is where Shaunda-Lee learned to open her heart and home to young girls in danger and in distress. When Shaunda-Lee moved into her first home she always brought in young ladies in distress. So it is not surprising that her passion for these ladies runs deep. Growing up with a Monster as her father, she understood the importance of a safe haven and why they are necessary.

"My goal is to redirect Millennial and Y-gen traffic so to speak. Educate them properly and encourage them to share this knowledge with friends, and family and with their own daughters to continue to save lives through prevention."

"Our Daughters Deserve The Best, The Time For Settling IS Over!"